RESCUE

Dr. Tim Buchman

RESCUE

A Surgeon's Memoir of Life, Death, and the Calling to Save Lives

CHESTNUT HALL
BOOKS

This book is a memoir. It reflects the author's personal experiences and opinions. It is not intended as medical advice. Readers should consult qualified health professionals for medical guidance.

Certain identifying details have been changed to protect patient confidentiality.

The views expressed in this work are solely those of the author and do not represent those of any affiliated institutions.

Published by Chestnut Hall Books
Atlanta, Georgia
www.drtimbuchman.com

Paperback ISBN: 979-8-9951328-0-6
eBook (Kindle) ISBN: 979-8-9951328-1-3

First edition

10 9 8 7 6 5 4 3 2

Cover design by Bethany Williams and Tammy Kling

Printed in the United States of America

CHESTNUT HALL
BOOKS

Table of Contents

Introduction

This is a memoir. That sounds straightforward until you ask the next question: what, exactly, is a memoir?

It is not an autobiography. It makes no pretense of completeness. It does not promise a full accounting, a comprehensive timeline, or a tidy inventory of accomplishments and affiliations. Nor is it the familiar genre of history told from a privileged perch - the recounting of some famous event seen through the equally famous eyes of someone who, by name alone, is assumed to matter more than the rest of us.

A memoir is something quieter and, in a way, more demanding. It is an exercise in introspection. It is the discipline of choosing: moments and episodes that adhered - scenes that would not fully leave, that kept returning unbidden, that continued to reverberate long after the immediate urgency had passed. A memoir does not claim, "This is everything." It says instead, "These are the points where the surface broke and the deeper structure showed itself."

I have come to think of it the way winter reveals a tree.

In the summer and fall we admire the lushness of leaves, the fullness of shade, the effortless impression of vitality. We notice the rhythms of tree life: birds nesting, squirrels negotiating impossible branches, the bright percussion of woodpeckers by day, the more secret movements of owls by night. The tree feels like abundance made visible. And because it is so visibly alive, the architecture and flows that make it possible - the trunk's strength, the branching decisions, the sap's quiet insistence - are merely assumed. We enjoy the canopy; we rarely study what sustains it.

Then winter arrives. The leaves release. The canopy thins to honesty. And what becomes visible is not merely absence but structure: the trunk, the branching, the old nests held in place by sticky geometry. You can see where storms once tested the tree. You can see the scar that didn't kill it. You can see the limb that chose a direction and never reconsidered. Even the emptiness has meaning; it outlines what was there, and what will return.

A memoir performs that winter work. It clears away the lushness - not to diminish the life that was lived, but to expose the framework that carried it. It shows the trunk and enough branches, enough nests, enough evidence of passage, that someone who looks carefully will not see only this tree - this cellulose skeleton covered in aged bark - but something larger and strangely familiar.

These trees are not identical, and yet they are recognizably of a shared world.

In the revealed architecture of one person's life, a reader may glimpse the outline of another: a neighbor's, a friend's, a parent's, a child's. Sometimes, unmistakably, their own. Not the details - the names, the dates, the particular streets and institutions - but the shape: the places where pressure concentrated, where responsibility demanded something costly, where a decision was made without certainty, where a loss left a visible line, where endurance began to look like character.

That is my hope behind these stories.

They are drawn from a life of rescue - episodes of urgency and improvisation, of failure and learning, of hard-won competence and the occasional grace of outcomes that feel like gifts. But they are not offered as a display, and certainly not as a monument.

This is not an invitation to gaze upon my tree in winter as if it were exotic or exemplary.

It is, instead, an invitation - perhaps even a permission - to look at another tree and then to recognize your own.

It is an invitation to see, in the exposed structure of a rescuer's life, the deep architecture that makes any life possible: the branches we inherited, the branches we chose, the nests we tended without quite naming them, the scars we carry, the quiet flows that keep us standing when the season strips away what once looked like certainty.

If this book succeeds, it will not be because you learn my chronology. It will be because you find your own questions rising as you read - and because you begin, in your own way, to see your trunk and your branches more clearly.

A single winter tree is truly revealing. But it is also, if we are honest, a convenient illusion. It is an illusion because rescue does not happen in the life of one person the way a tree stands alone in a field.

Rescue happens in a grove. It happens in weather. It happens inside a landscape we did not plant by ourselves, soil we inherited, storms we could not schedule, seasons that arrive without permission. And when winter exposes the architecture, what you begin to see is not only one trunk and its branches, but the interlacing of many: roots in conversation underground, limbs braided by proximity, nests that migrate from one tree to another, and the invisible corridors of wind that carry both danger and relief.

That is what our work of rescue is like.

This book is for you.

This book is for anyone who wants our insiders' perspective on rescue, or validation of the work we do.

We speak as if rescue belongs to a single rescuer because a story needs a face and a pair of hands. We tell ourselves the monomythology of the lone capable figure - decisive, calm, competent, singular - because the mind wants a clean narrative: a problem, a hero, an outcome. But in the lived world of healthcare, heroism is rarely solitary. It is distributed. It is layered. It is threaded through a hundred small acts most people never see and almost no one applauds.

The patient meets a clinician at the bedside. That encounter feels like the whole truth because it is the most human truth. But behind it - beneath it - is an entire ecology of preparation, vigilance, and constraint.

There is the voice on the phone who knows what to ask when the caller cannot speak clearly. There is the dispatcher who makes time do impossible things. There is the paramedic who chooses a road and a rhythm of compressions and a dose, and who carries a stranger's life in the space between intersections. There is the nurse who recognizes a change before it has a name. The respiratory therapist who senses fatigue in a chest long before a monitor can prove it. The pharmacist who catches the dose that would have become a tragedy. The lab technologist who runs toward the specimen, not away from it. The radiology technologist who positions a body that cannot help itself. The environmental services worker who restores the room to safety so the next suffering person does not inherit the last one's microbes. The clerk who finds the missing number. The transporter who moves the patient as if moving them were itself a form of care because it is.

And beyond those faces, beyond the immediate circle of the room - there are the structures that determine whether rescue is even possible: staffing models, training cultures, handoff norms, the quality of a supply chain, the reliability of equipment, the design of a pager system, the clarity of escalation pathways, the safety of a workplace, the willingness of good leaders to see and to speak and to tell the truth about capacity.

There are administrators who decide what is funded and what is deferred. There are policies that shape time at the bedside as much as any stethoscope does. There are budgets that become, in practice, moral documents. There are leaders who do not touch a patient and yet profoundly touch the conditions under which patients live or die.

You know these people.
You are likely one of them.

You cannot read these stories - truly read them - without feeling this. Even the episodes that appear to revolve around one decision or one pair of hands are never only that. The room is full, even when it looks empty. The rescue is plural, even when the narrative pronoun is singular.

And this is where the book's central claim begins to clarify itself: you cannot have successes without failures and lessons - not as an individual, and not as an organization.

In the clinical world, failure is not merely a private embarrassment; it is a signal. Sometimes it is a signal that a human being reached their limits of knowledge, attention, stamina, or skill. Sometimes it is a signal that the system made predictable error likely: too many patients, too few hands, too much noise, not enough rest, unclear ownership, a culture that punishes escalation, a reluctance to admit uncertainty. Sometimes it is both at once - the human and the system tangled together, each amplifying the other.

That is why these stories move between triumph and fracture, between competence and regret, between gratitude and grief. I have not arranged them to perform drama. I have cast them to tell the truth: rescue is not a straight line, and it is not clean. It is iterative. It is communal. It is costly. It is, at times, unbearably beautiful precisely because it occurs in the same world that contains loss.

If this book leaves you tender, that tenderness is not weakness. It is recognition.

It means you have begun to see what rescuers often spend years trying not to see too clearly: that we are dependent creatures, bound together by physiology and time and chance; that our best work is never only ours; that our worst moments never belong to one person alone; and that the distance between catastrophe and recovery is crossed by teams - sometimes coordinated brilliantly, sometimes held together by improvisation and sheer moral will.

So yes, this is a memoir. It is one tree in winter.

But it is also a map of a forest.

It is written for those who run toward alarms and for those who quietly ensure the alarms are heard. It is written for clinicians and first responders, and for the leaders and organizations who decide every day - whether the work will be sustainable, whether truth will be speakable, whether help will arrive in time, whether the next generation will be mentored instead of consumed.

It begins with a question that sounds individual, even private:

Why am I on this path?

And it inevitably becomes the only question that can bear the full weight of the work:

Why are <u>we</u> on this path?

The pages that follow are my attempt to answer - not with doctrine, not with completeness, but with scenes that stayed. Scenes that exposed the trunk. Scenes that reveal how rescue actually happens: across roles, across shifts, across years; through failures that become lessons; through lessons that become the conditions of success; through the stubborn, luminous truth that no one wants to learn the hard way and yet all of us eventually must:

You are not alone.

No one rescues alone.

Now, let us begin.

Prologue - The Call to Rescue

The world imagines our days and nights through on-screen spectacle. Flashing lights, shouted orders, expected miracles realized in this week's episode of a hit TV show. Such is the imagined life of a first responder, an emergency physician, an ICU nurse, a trauma surgeon, an EMT or paramedic, policeman or sheriff's deputy. You know who they are.

You know who you are.

Our work starts long before and ends long after anyone is watching.

It often begins in darkness.

A pager. A siren. The rush of adrenaline. We move before thinking, because that is how the body protects the mind, grabbing bag and badge and purpose.

How do you enter the maelstrom?

Are you the EMT at the curve in the road, your breath clouding as you kneel beside twisted metal?

Are you the ED nurse catching the never-ending flow of arrivals on foot, by car, by ambulance, by helicopter?

Are you the trauma surgeon deciding whether you can pause long enough to get a CT scan or whether you need to head directly to the OR?

Are you standing guard in the ICU, wondering what mixture of blood components and vasopressors might yield stability from the physiological chaos that arrived 5 minutes ago?

Are you the palliative care professional trying to make sense of shattered dreams for the patient and the family?

Your title, credentials, and location might be different from your colleagues'. Your shared imperative remains: "I will make this better."

Life is metered in twelve-hour segments that stretch into forever. Sleep comes in fragments, meals in gulps. Weekends, birthdays, holidays are "in concept only." The people who love you learn to live around your absence, even when you are physically present.

You have been exposed to pathogens, to rage, to grief so dense it feels radioactive.

You have been accused, adored, ignored, and sometimes assaulted.

You have made impossible choices from incomplete information, and you live with them long after everyone else has gone home.

You don the mask of calm that hides your fear, because fear has no place at the bedside—except that it always does, in secret, as vigilance.

You have buried colleagues lost not to physical trauma but inexorable burnout that culminates in addiction, descent into despair, and violent escape from this world.

You carry the ghost of the child you couldn't save and of the patient you saved who no longer wanted saving.

You hope that you were good enough, whatever that means.

The fatigue seeps into your bones. Your life expectancy is truncated by stress. Empathy is harder to find. Yet every morning—or night—or both—you show up to answer that first, next call.

Yours is not a job. Jobs end when the shift does.

Yours might be a profession; at heart, a covenant.

Your work is a promise you make to strangers. It is a promise you keep at great personal cost.

For many of you, it remains a calling, an inescapable tinnitus demanding your service that reverberates through every siren, alarm, sign-out, and farewell.

This book is about you, your call to rescue, and what lies beneath your commitment.

What it gives.

What it takes.

What it reveals.

Before we go further—before our stories, the science, our search for balance—we pause for the query that matters most, the one that binds all rescuers across every corridor of care.

Find a mirror, look into your eyes, and ask yourself this single question:

"Why am I on this path?"

1 - LEARNING TO LEARN

My first course in medical school was Anatomy 301 and it began with a lesson I did not yet know how to name: humility. It arrived quietly, without fanfare, as the realization that I was wholly unprepared for the journey I was undertaking.

I had neatly sidestepped biology in high school. In college, I tested out of the required courses, choosing instead the comforts of physics and the clean precision of circuits, lenses, and magnets. Nothing in those carefully structured experiences resembled the ten-week immersion in gross anatomy I was about to face.

There were six of us in the summer anatomy class, all MD–PhD students. The regular class of one hundred MD-only students would not begin until fall. Our professor was a world-renowned scholar and paleontologist. He met with us every day.

Week 1, Day 1: we were issued our dissection kits, introduced to our cadavers, and instructed to begin with the right shoulder and arm. Music stands held our atlases. The sharp smell of formalin perfused the lab, permeated our coats, and became part of our dreams.

I let my partner take the scalpel while I hovered with the textbook, trying to match color plates with what lay before us. The pages were crisp and labeled; the arm in my hands was uniformly brown and decidedly not. I could not yet see what I needed to see.

By Friday afternoon, "fake it 'til you make it" had vanished. The professor's oral reviews were unforgiving. One student at a time, on someone else's cadaver, he exposed structures and expected us to name them, describe their function, and trace their course.

"Mr. Buchman," he said, "where has your brain been the past five days and four nights?"

I had no answer. His verdict was simple and accurate: F.

He asked me to wait until he had finished with the others. Then he opened his office door and gestured me inside, a gesture as old as apprenticeship itself: sit down; we need to talk.

"You seem to be struggling."

I admitted as much.

"So…you've never dissected a fish, a frog, a fetal pig. Yet here you are trying to learn the architecture of the human body."

Correct.

"And you are attempting to master this by memorizing the textbook."

Also correct.

He was not unkind. He was simply unblinking.

"I can more or less guarantee you will fail the course if you continue this way."

In that moment, I met one of the first mirrors of my training, the honest one, the one that shows you exactly where you stand before earning the right to stand elsewhere. Humility, again.

He moved to his bookshelf and retrieved a volume.

"You cannot create logic from facts. Without logic, you will drown. And you do not yet have the logic of embryology, or comparative anatomy, or physiology on which the facts must hang. Yet here you are trying to become a doctor."

Then, after another moment's thought:

"This weekend, you are not to open your textbook. Take this. Study Unit 6. See me in the lab Monday at 9 a.m."

The book was Case Studies in Anatomy—a first edition inscribed to him by its author, Ernest Lachman. These were stories of patients and pathology, of people in need and doctors called to act. I did not have the language for it then, but this was my earliest glimpse of the rescuer's formation: anatomy not as structure but as the foundation upon which suffering is recognized and care is imagined and help is rendered.

On Monday, he was waiting. He uncovered a new and unfamiliar arm.

"Tell me what this structure is," he said, "and why a doctor should know it."

My answers were imperfect but sound. He reclaimed his book (it was inscribed to him, after all) and voiced that a copy was available in the bookstore. Once again, he saw what I needed before I did.

The next nine weeks were difficult. I finished with a hard-earned C—far from glorious, yet honorable in its own way, especially given that he had not awarded an A in nearly a decade. I survived. No one has ever asked about my grade in Gross Anatomy.

But humility had done its quiet work: that first week's failure did not end me; it instructed me.

At the end of the course, he summoned me.

"You were utterly unprepared," he began.

I agreed.

"But you never quit. You earned your C."

He paused.

"One of the teaching assistants for the MD-only class has fallen ill. The position is open. I think you should take it. Teaching will advance your learning. Preparing each day, you will discover what you do not know."

It was my first formal step into apprenticeship. I was no longer merely learning from a master. I graduated to learning by helping others climb the same steep path. Teaching required me to understand, not recite; to see, not merely name.

Ten weeks later, at the end of my teaching assistantship, he called me in once more.

"You now command the basics of anatomy. Your charges are better prepared for the quizzes than most."

Faint praise, but faint praise in training carries more weight than flattery. It means you have progressed.

"The summer C stands," he said. "But in the fall, each of your students earned my top grade—B. You have both a talent and a passion for teaching anatomy. All you need is the opportunity and the logic."

Coda

His lessons remained long after our paths diverged: facts without logic are useless; learning requires finding the logic; teaching requires communicating it. These were not just academic principles. They were early lessons in how rescuers are shaped: through humility, through apprenticeship, through the slow transformation of confusion into competence, and competence into service.

A quarter-century later, as a mid-career academic surgeon, I was summoned to the Dean's office.

"The students want to be in your operating room, even those who don't have any interest in surgery." He paused. "They say you make anatomy come alive."

"Each year," he continued, "the honor of administering the Hippocratic Oath goes to the professor selected by the graduating class as their best teacher. I cannot recall the last time they chose a surgeon."

He paused again.

"Congratulations."

Rescuer In The Mirror

I did not walk into Anatomy 301 unprepared by accident. I walked in unprepared because I was counting credits and counting dollars, and placement exams looked like a rational shortcut. The course made a different kind of accounting unavoidable.

What stung was not the grade. It was being seen clearly by a master who could name the gap between what I wanted to be and what I had actually done to prepare. That humiliation became useful only when I stopped treating it as shame and started treating it as method: find the logic first, then hang facts on it, then test the logic at the table.

The deeper surprise was that I did not truly learn anatomy until I had to teach it. Competence became transmissible only after it became organized.

My advice: when you fail under scrutiny, do not argue with the mirror. Convert humiliation into apprenticeship. Aim less for brief brilliance and more for durable reliability, the kind that keeps showing up and keeps getting better.

Mirror question: Where are you mistaking shame for a verdict instead of a signal to apprentice?

2 - REDIRECTED

Fortunately, my embarrassment in Anatomy 301 was the worst of it. Microbiology, biochemistry, physiology and later pathology were all somewhat familiar and easier to organize. After the two pre-clinical years, my classmates continued on with their white coat ceremony and onto the wards. We MD-PhD types (our classmates referred to us by a vaguely derogatory, alliterative "mud-fuds") split off into our research years.

In my younger days, I had both a hankering and some aptitude for chemistry. I had earned my master's degree in organic chemistry, passed my PhD "prelims", a rite of passage that included a written submission and an oral examination about a project meant to occupy me for a few years. But I woke up one day realizing that I would become a good chemist, but never a great one. I lacked the necessary passion, or at least the lab's vaporized carbon compounds lacked the capacity to stir that passion.

I confessed as much to my PhD advisor, who took it rather well. He listened patiently, thanked me for my candor, and then wrote down the name of a man whose lecture he had recently attended, someone he thought I might be a fit for.

I called and arranged an interview. The man was the Chair of the Committee on Virology, someone who devoted his life to the study of a single family of viruses. We spoke for perhaps a half hour, and then he asked me, "Which interests you most DNA, RNA, or protein?" These were rather separate territories in the mid-1970s, and I responded, "DNA." He, too, wrote a name on a piece of paper, told me this was one of his post-doctoral fellows, and that I should learn from him.

Graduate students learn many things, and in many ways. There is science at the bench. How to plan an experiment, how to think about controls and procedures and what could go wrong. How to embrace all of the results, especially the unexpected anomalous one. How to frame the experiment and its outcome into the endless conversation of meaning that scientists refer to as "theory" but is as close to truth as we will ever know.

The other thing I learned was that writing, particularly scientific writing, was both a necessary skill and an unforgiving mistress.

I drafted my first report, typed it up, and dropped it off with his secretary. A few days later, she called me and told me that the Chair wanted to see me. No, not right away, she said. Not at the lab. At his house. Tonight. 8 p.m. From her voice, I could tell that meant being on the doorstep at 7:55 p.m.

I rang the bell. The door opened to a petite woman, a legal librarian who had married the Chair four years before I was born. Her faint smile suggested I was not the first to ever answer such summons. She pointed towards a door and invited me to descend.

The Chair's home office was decidedly different from the one at the lab. He sat behind an aircraft carrier-sized desk. Behind him on the wall were his name badges from every conference he had ever attended. There was a white long-haired cat in his lap, and he was stroking it Blofeld-like.

He and the cat both looked at me.

"There are a yellow pad and a pencil on the desk. Pick it up. Please."

Manners, always.

He and the cat sat back in his chair. He spoke steadily for the next half hour or so. I transcribed furiously, double spaced and large letters so I would be able to go back and make sense of the scribble.

When he was done, I realized that he had dictated a perfect paper based on my imperfect data and even more imperfect draft.

The cat did not blink.

"Go type it up and have it for my secretary tomorrow."

Before I scuttled back up the stairs, I had to ask.

"How did you do that?"

He let the question hang before answering: "This was your first. It was not mine."

Years later I emerged from the lab somewhat better at science and at writing, PhD in hand, ready to return and begin my clinical years as the most junior member of the bedside team. It was obvious to even the most casual observer that my future lay in internal medicine, with a subspecialty in infectious disease. What else would a virologist do, after all?

My first student rotation was on the pediatric service, where I loved the kids but—never having been the parent of a sick child—hated the moms. I learned the basics of hospital life, endured the clinics, and passed by the pediatric ICU from time to time, catching sight of cathode ray tubes displaying green numbers I somehow recalled from physiology half a decade earlier.

The plan, then, was to rotate through surgery to "get ready for medicine." There would be some mandatory time in the OR, but perhaps most of it could be avoided.

My first night on the Gold surgical service, an older woman with a cancerous breast that would be amputated the next day tolerated this medical student laboring through her history and a clumsy physical examination. I was perhaps halfway through the latter when the chief resident stopped in and told me I was needed in the OR. I briefly objected on the grounds that I hadn't fulfilled my current responsibility—only to be silenced by an unblinking glare that needed no translation: my hind end, along with the rest of me, should already have been moving.

I scrubbed in as the third assistant. There were four of us at the operating table. The attending, a young gastrointestinal surgeon who would later become famous as a world's expert on inflammatory bowel disease, and the chief resident were deep in the abdomen of a woman who had been stabbed in a domestic dispute. I was there along with the intern to hold retractors—the "learning sticks" of which medical students are not terribly fond—and to watch, and to listen.

Some memories of structures from the Anatomy 301 days bubbled to the surface. More were prodded loose by questions from the attending surgeon, to which my answers earned approving grunts (always preferred to more caustic commentary). At any rate, the patient looked quite sick in the recovery area. Surprisingly, though, she got better in a few days and went home. I never saw her again.

I did, however, go back to the operating room.

The most senior attending on the service—the Boss—was a Korean Conflict veteran who now waged war against colon cancer. He, too, offered learning sticks, and questions, and acknowledging grunts.

His patients also got better.

Mostly.

One evening toward the end of my rotation on his Gold service, I was getting ready to go home, having been on call and up most of the previous night, when I learned that a patient of the Boss from the prior week had returned to the ED. I had done one of those histories and physicals I mentioned so I went down to see her on my way out. The intern was preparing to wheel her to the radiology suite, where she was to undergo an enema with water-soluble contrast to check the integrity of the anastomosis that the boss and the resident had laboriously constructed ten days earlier. The intern had another patient to see and asked if I would take the patient up to radiology. The intern would be just a minute, he said.

An hour and a half later, she and I were still in the radiology suite when the Boss came in. The intern was nowhere in sight.

The Boss was resplendent in tuxedo and cowboy boots: one of his larger-than-life surgical looks. He eyed me and said, "Weren't you supposed to be home tonight?" That was quickly followed by, "Page the intern…now."

I did.

The intern showed up a couple of minutes later. They had words, and the intern's face turned the color of his vaguely white coat.

The Boss looked at the studies, pronounced the anastomosis intact, and then crooked a finger.

Follow me.

We went to his office. He opened a drawer in his desk while asking me what I planned to do with my life.

"Internal medicine, sir. Infectious disease."

A bottle of bourbon appeared. Really. And two glasses. He poured us each a finger. Maybe two.

He drank. I spluttered. Bourbon is a bit of an acquired taste and skill, and at that moment I had neither.

"When you finally realize that you are a surgeon, come see me. Now go home."

My next rotation was on the internal medicine service. It was supposed to be glorious. I hated it. We did nothing but dole out pills. We managed this and that, but we never really made anyone better.

A few weeks later, I called the Boss's secretary, a grandmotherly type who answered the phone before the second ring.

I explained who I was and why I was calling.

She replied that she had been told to expect my call, and that there was an opening on Tuesday at 5 p.m. and not to be late.

I was there at 4:55.

Rescuer In The Mirror

Most of us begin training convinced we know our destination. I did. I left chemistry not because I could not be good at it, but because I needed to make a difference I could feel—and so could the people around me.

The pivot was not insight; it was mentorship. A senior surgeon saw the mismatch between my declared plan and my lived response to the work, and he named it plainly. Letting go of a prior identity can feel like betrayal—of a lab, of a mentor, even of your own past—yet the cost of staying on the wrong path is higher and paid in quieter currency.

My advice: let your path redirect you before it breaks you. Ask two questions early and often: What work gives me energy? What work makes me useful? Then ask the people who know you well what they see, and listen without defending your first draft of yourself.

Mirror question: What are you still calling "my plan" that your own behavior has already outgrown?

3 - SCHRÖDINGER'S CAT

Medical students take national examinations in common. The process of choosing a specialty and matching into a program is a rite of passage that culminates around the Ides of March of the final year in medical school. In those days, in the early Spring of 1980, the fates of tens of thousands of physicians-to-be were decided by a faceless mainframe computer located somewhere (no one quite knew the precise location—security and all that) in Evanston, IL. After costly travel and endless interviews, students would prepare their preference list, programs would prepare their preference lists, and the algorithm loosed upon them. For some weeks the computer knew, and the results were delivered in sealed envelopes to medical schools from Miami to Honolulu.

On the appointed day, at noon on the east coast, and 9 am on the west coast, and some ungodly hour in Hawai'i (medical school in paradise comes with at least this one minor inconvenience), there was a rush to the table to find the envelope with one's name and find out where the next years of one's life would be spent. Some cheered, some cried, and many opened and stared in silence.

The Boss had forbidden me to rank Chicago where I had spent the past 9 years. You have to see the world, he said. So I joined the ranks of those looking for cheap flights, cheaper hotels, and a suit that would not wrinkle. I visited the programs, terrified by one, disappointed in another, mildly insulted by a third. The fourth, though, seemed welcoming enough. I put it at the top of my list, albeit with some trepidation. More on that in a moment.

At 11 a.m. in Chicago on Match Day I joined the run to the table and tore open the envelope. I still have the slip of paper that told me, five decades ago, that I had been selected to be a Halsted Surgical Intern at the Johns Hopkins Hospital in Baltimore.

Day 1 Intern

In late June, I pointed the car east and a little south. A few days later, I found myself at orientation in a basement auditorium, the Tilghman Room, on the Johns Hopkins medical campus in East Baltimore.

There were twenty new surgical interns—a few insiders, the rest hopeful strangers like me—shuffled into the rows. The three new Hopkins surgical "Super Chiefs"—technically the Assistant Chiefs of all Hopkins surgery—strode into the room, resplendent in crisp white coats, each carrying a stack of three-ring binders.

The first intoned, "You'll find inside your schedules, regulations, and the Hopkins handbook. The index card has the pager numbers of everyone on the housestaff. Your pager is clipped to that index card."

The second continued, "You get two sets of uniforms—white pants, short jackets. One to wear after the first is splattered. Bleach them at every wash. Keep the pager index card in the breast pocket so you'll always know where it is.

The third told us the details of our hard-won match. "Your job is to keep "the book"— your service's record of every patient's vital signs, labs, X-rays. If it's not written, it never happened. Don't ever let the book out of your grasp. Ever."

The first chief walked to the chalkboard. "Your schedule is the Halsted schedule. You'll be here every day. Your first week begins Saturday morning. You'll leave Monday night when the work is done. The other intern will stay Monday night. You'll return Tuesday morning, go home Wednesday evening. Show up Thursday morning and work through Saturday morning. The next week inverts. It has always been this way, and it will always be this way. Eat when you can, sleep when you can, it's up to you to find that time."

The second chief delivered the news we all knew was coming but didn't quite want to accept. "You transitional interns know your future. For the nine of you categorical surgical interns, this is a pyramidal program. Look left. Look right. Only one of the three of you will finish and stand up here in five years' time."

Translation: we had a one in three chance of standing where they were five years downrange. Otherwise, well…no one wanted to think about that. They told us that we would be scrutinized throughout the internship and told at the beginning of the second year whether there would be a third and fourth and fifth and sixth year.

Then we were shoo'ed out. "Find your service at 5:00 a.m. tomorrow. Good luck."

That night, I lay awake in an unfamiliar room, new uniforms on the bureau, two alarm clocks each set for 4:00 on either side of the bed, the pager a foot away. Thunder rumbled in the distance, countered by the wail of an ambulance.

A Year Later

The year passed quickly, more quickly than I expected. Except for two weeks' vacation and two days at either Thanksgiving or Christmas or New Years (assigned, not chosen) it was non-stop pre-ops, protocols, and long hours holding retractors while those above us worked their magic in the surgical field. When we were stuck on the ward, we wished we were in the operating room; when in the OR, we fretted about the admissions waiting for "H and Ps"—medical histories, physical exams, admitting orders, and blood draws—all the interns' work.

Now, in the second year, our anxiety had shifted. We all wondered who among our intern class would be invited to stay and who would "pyramid out", hoping to find a spot in some small community hospital or perhaps change careers to something less toxic.

One evening that first week of the second year, I signed the service out to the new intern just after six with the traditional admonition: "Keep 'em alive 'til five-oh-five."

Then I crossed the street, popped a TV dinner in the oven, pulled a Coca-Cola from the fridge. The food made me sleepy: I set my alarms and crawled into bed just after sunset.

I woke to the scream of my pager on the nightstand:

"Dr. Buchman, report to OR 2. Dr. Buchman, you are needed in OR 2."

I pulled on a fresh pair of scrubs, crossed the street, bounded up the stairs, and scrubbed in. The newly minted Assistant Chief of Service (he had been in the role 3 days), Aaron, and one of the senior residents were head-down, trying to control bleeding. A medical student held one retractor. Aaron called for a "Big Rich", an instrument resembling a garden hoe used to lift the abdominal wall and expose the deepest reaches of the abdomen. As I pulled, I glanced up at the clock: 1:45 a.m.

We pulled for two hours. Eventually, the bleeding came under control, the bullet holes found and repaired, the cavity washed out with buckets of saline. It was time to close.

Aaron turned to me.

"There's a bowel obstruction in the ED. You can scrub out and get the H and P done."

"Can't the intern do that?"

"What are you talking about? You are the intern."

I hesitated. "No. Bob, the new intern, is on tonight."

Aaron looked momentarily confused.

"You were on last night. What are you doing here?"

The circulating nurse, God bless her, overheard us.

"You told me to page Dr. Buchman to the OR. I did. He came and he's been holding that retractor for you the entire case."

Aaron muttered an expletive, then:

"Go home."

"Aaron, rounds start in an hour. The new intern's still trying to figure out how to get from one ward to another. I'll make sure he gets the H and P done on the guy in the ED."

I did just that, then went up to the locker room, showered, and shaved. A full day of clinic lay ahead, and I was sure the bowel-obstruction patient would end up in the OR soon enough. I found Bob on the ward getting the admission settled. I grabbed a donut and coffee and headed for rounds.

The next few days were busy, but not crazy busy. The obstruction did go to the OR, along with the usual emergency lineup: two appendectomies, a gallbladder, a wet gangrene, a diabetic abscess. The Friday elective list included two breast biopsies and an umbilical hernia. What would have seemed impossibly overwhelming a year earlier had become business as usual.

By Saturday morning—Bob's turn on call—I was more than ready for a real sleep. I left him the chores except for the woman with the drained thigh abscess; I knew the geography of the wound, and it was going to be painful enough for her without having a new intern fumbling through.

I had just pulled off my gloves when the pager screeched:

"Six-Oh-Six-Six, please call Six-Oh-Six-Six."

The office of the Chairman of Surgery.

I found a phone. He answered on the second ring.

"Tim, please come down to the office now."

Now I was wide awake.

I thought of Schrödinger's Cat, its superpositioned ears perking up (and also not) sensing that someone was opening the box; that opening that would paradoxically seal its fate. Would I be one of the chosen to stay on, or would I be told to find a post elsewhere?

I splashed cold water on my face, ran a comb through my hair, and put on a clean pair of scrubs. The shower and shave would have to wait.

Down the stairs, past decades of photographs of Halsted Chief Residents staring back at me. I steadied myself, took a deep breath, walked past his secretary's station into his office, and chose to remain standing at a respectful (and hopefully non-smellable) distance.

The Chairman looked up from his desk.

"Close the door, please."

My heart was hammering.

"What are your plans for the next few years?" he asked.

I hesitated. "If it's all the same to you, sir, I'd really like to stay on and become a Halsted Assistant Chief of Service."

He looked at me over the top of his glasses. A ghost of a smile appeared.

"I think that can be arranged."

Then: "Not a word to anyone until I make a general announcement in ten days. No one. And leave the door open on your way out. Congratulations, you've earned it."

I mumbled something like thank you and somehow made it back across the street and into bed.

When I woke, it was dark. I opened the refrigerator, reached for a Coca-Cola, and grabbed a National Bohemian instead. If any day deserved a Natty Bo, surely this one qualified.

I crawled back into bed. No alarms needed. Tomorrow was mine.

I reached over to turn my pager off … and stopped.

No Halsted Super Chief was ever unreachable.

I wouldn't be, either.

Somewhere in the distance thunder rumbled and an ambulance wailed.

This time I had no trouble falling asleep.

Rescuer In The Mirror

Training is uncertainty made physical: incomplete information, high stakes, and judgment required before comfort arrives. The Halsted schedule was extreme, but the deeper demand was psychological: be reachable, be accountable, and learn in public.

Constant availability has a price. So does its absence. The point is not martyrdom; it is formation. You learn from patients, not books, and you learn fastest when the data are incomplete and the mirror is the only place to find the next decision.

My advice: treat training as an anchor, not as an assault. Do not romanticize hardship, but do not flee challenge either. Protect sleep and relationships where you can—and when the flying moments arrive, improve them rather than avoid them.

Mirror question: What part of "being reachable" are you resisting—and is it boundary setting, or avoidance?

4 - FUEL

The internship was lived. It also had to be survived.

Napoleon Bonaparte remarked, "*An army marches on its stomach*"; rescuers continue this tradition of essential alimentation. Novitiates learn the truth of three time-honored commandments of surgical training: "Eat when you can, sleep when you can, and do not mess with the pancreas during an operation." Of these, the most important is the first: *eat when you can.*

Surgical interns stream into the hospital during darkness. In summer, they might see dusk after one or two nights on call while staggering home. Between these times—between histories and physical exams, between holding retractors in the operating room, and between assembling at 3 PM outside the hematology lab to rifle through the wood box containing the results of the morning draw—they forage.

A young attending not so far removed from his own intern years would occasionally bring two dozen Dunkin' Donuts to the break room on Sunday mornings.

There were heady noontimes when a pharmaceutical rep put on a "drug lunch", an unholy deal involving a sandwich and a bag of chips in exchange for 'learning 'about a newly patented antibiotic.

Towards evening, our sensitive noses could smell hot pizza three wards distant.

Food mattered.

Imagine David Attenborough narrating: *"Here we see the surgical interns in their habitat, one eye on the clock and the other on their clipboard, noses trained to sniff out morsels of food. The main cafeteria is six floors down. The OR cafeteria has closed. An unopened packet of saltine crackers lies isolated at the nearby nurses 'station..."*

Day becomes evening. Vending machines beckon, ignored by the intern as he hurries to fetch another two units of packed red blood cells from the blood bank for the patient just transferred to the surgical intensive care unit on Halsted 7. The units are checked, the blood is hung, and I steal a glance into the ICU break room.

There! On the table! A family has brought a basket of high-calorie, nutritionally empty treats. I rush toward it, only to realize that it is an empty mirage. The basket has been there for four hours, and the half-life of such baskets is around 26 minutes in a busy ICU. (There was that one exception when the family of a renowned "diet guru" brought his branded treats to the ICU. That half-life was measured in days. His company went bankrupt.)

It is now approaching one o'clock in the morning. There is no reason for any human to be awake at this hour. Last night's partiers should be home in bed; the earliest morning workers should still be dreaming of the day to come. For us interns, though, it is our time.

Here again is imagined David Attenborough: *"They glance at the clock. As the hour approaches three, they move, sharing some secret signal. They go to the corridor, to the elevator, down to the corridor that leads to the Monument Street door to the hospital. They stop short at the lights that blaze from the corridor's west side. They have reached their feeding ground."*

The Corridor Café. Or, as the interns called it, The Coronary Café.

There is a young man behind the counter, not so different in age from us interns, but from a different world. He feeds us to support his family, working a second job while his young wife, her mom, and their child sleep. He knows us, our habits, our timing. He knows that we will descend upon him in the minutes before official closing.

He is ready. In the hour before, he has hand-dipped a dozen milkshakes, mostly chocolate. (The first arrivals have their pick, while the stragglers will be grateful for whatever flavors are left.) Patties are placed in readiness, paper plates are loaded with buns and handfuls of chips. He knows we will come.

"Double cheeseburger with extra pickles, chocolate shake." He looks at me; he knows my order and the order of every other intern. We fish in our pockets for paper and coins. We sit, exchange stories, and look at our lists of the bits of remaining work. He smiles at us as he cleans the grill and dims the lights.

"Last one out, lock the door." He knows we will, because he knows that the other team will come in tonight, and we will return the night after.

It is still dark as we go to make one last check on the pre-ops. Soon, through the darkness, the incoming housestaff will arrive. We will assemble for pre-rounds, shuffling from one room to the next, reviewing what happened overnight.

These pre-rounds are the only moment of the day when our bellies are all full, and we can focus on the work at hand without hearing a stomach growl. We make our way from room to room, ward to ward, trying to finish in time for a cup of coffee before rounds begin in earnest.

I spy an unopened packet of saltines on a counter and slip it into my pocket.

"Eat when you can."

Field Notes

Fuel is not comfort; it is cognition. In rescue work, eating, hydrating, and resting are operational requirements before they are personal preferences.

Signal: Hunger, dehydration, and sleep debt show up first as irritability, tunnel vision, and brittle decision-making, long before they show up as obvious "fatigue."

Failure modes: Skipping meals, relying on vending-machine sugar, and normalizing sleeplessness create preventable cognitive errors and relationship erosion on shift.

Practice: Design your shifts the way you would design a resuscitation: plan fuel breaks, protect a minimum sleep block when possible, and use buddies (home and at work) to call you out when you are running empty.

DISCUSSION / WRITING PROMPTS (optional)

• What routines do you use to protect sleep, food, hydration, and movement during a typical shift week?

• If you had to work extended hours for weeks (disaster, surge, prolonged staffing failure), what would you change immediately to preserve judgment and safety?

5 - THE RESCUE CALLERS

Beneath the north side of Johns Hopkins Hospital, running parallel to Monument Street, lay a long corridor, broad enough for two gurneys to pass and quiet enough to hear the echo of a single step. In daylight, the basement corridor was lightly traveled; at night, almost deserted. Sometimes a stretcher emerged from the back door of the emergency department, escorted by nurses on their way to the ward or by the trauma team bound for the Blalock elevators and the operating room. Other times, those same elevators would open to a shrouded gurney, a lonely traveler on their journey to the morgue.

At the western end of that corridor, beside the service door of the Emergency Department, was an unmarked door. Behind it sat three women among telephones and microphones, their faces lit by the glow of incandescent bulbs and indicator lights of legacy switchboards. To me, they were Clotho, Lachesis, and Atropos—the Fates who spun, measured, and cut the threads of life. Their calm voices carried through every ward and corridor, summoning help, bearing witness, marking the boundaries between darkness and light.

In those pre-digital days—days and nights of overhead pages and voice pagers—it would happen that someone discovered a patient taking a turn for the worse, and a rescue had to be attempted. A shout to the unit clerk—"Call a code!"—and a special number would be dialed. The call rang down to that tiny room, and one of the three would answer, confirming the code and its location. Then she would reach for the guarded toggle, lift its cover, and cycle the switch.

GONG … GONG … GONG

The sound rolled through the hospital's concrete bones, felt as much as heard. Every ear listened for what would follow, each person hoping it was not their ward, their room, their patient. What came next was the thunder—a storm of footfalls racing toward whatever destination the Fates had announced.

This was a time before code teams, before choreographed responses. Whoever was near enough and brave enough would run. Someone took the airway; another began compressions; another searched for a vein. A nurse wheeled in the first generation electrocardiograph—forty pounds of metal on a rolling cart, hungry for an outlet. When she flipped the switch, the stylus would chatter across the narrow paper strip, tracing in black ink whatever syllables of a heart's rhythm it could find. Our decisions were made between those lines—compress or pause, shock or wait—each stroke of that stylus a measure in the music of survival.

Sometimes we won. The heart re-ignited, the stretcher rolled toward the ICU, and the ascent back into light began. But often we failed to rescue. The room grew still except for the AMBU bag's sigh. The most senior physician looked around at the faces of the rescuers, eyes silently asking: anyone have any more to offer?

Silence. A glance at the clock.

"Time of death: two twenty-three a.m."

We would step back, paper rustling, the appearance of the morgue pack: checklist, shroud, death certificate form. A little while later, a nurse and her patient would take that last elevator ride down, their slow descent through layers of light into that long corridor of final journeys.

I discovered the three ladies and their secret room, and the guarded toggle that made the GONGs, on a November day in 1980. Our pagers ran on AA batteries, and mine had gone weak. Normally, there were spares at the OR desk or in the ICU, but I happened to be in the ED when I noticed the signal fading. I went out the back door, walked ten feet, and knocked on the unmarked door.

It opened. The woman at the middle desk—her hair henna over white—read my name badge and recited my pager number before I could speak.

"Nice to put a face to a number, Hon," she said. Hon was a term of endearment peculiar to twentieth-century Baltimore. "Happy Thanksgiving. What brings you here?"

"A battery," I said. "May I please have a battery?"

She smiled and opened a drawer neatly lined with rows of AAs. "Here you go, Hon. Keep spares in your pocket. Those little beepers always die when you need them most."

All three women smiled as she pressed the battery into my hand. "Don't be a stranger. Come visit!"

I did.

From time to time, I stopped by for replacements, sometimes bringing a small bag of penny candy from the gift shop. The years passed. Before leaving for my Shock Trauma fellowship, I stopped in to tell them I'd be away for a while.

When I returned as an attending surgeon to build the Adult Trauma Service, one of my first tasks was to create a system of voice pagers for the team—two calls only: Alpha Trauma Team for the gravest cases, Bravo Trauma Team for those outwardly stable. It meant another meeting with the paging operators. I walked down the familiar tunnel and knocked on the unmarked door.

A new face appeared. I asked about my old friend, the one of the henna-over-white hair.

"She retired two months ago," the others said. "But we knew you'd be back, and your fresh battery's waiting."

I took it, thanked them, and turned it over in my hand, this small cylinder of stored promise. The hospital above had changed—new faces, new systems, new urgency—but the quiet current that bound it together still hummed behind that door. Energy passed from one set of hands to another, keeping the wheel of rescue turning, from darkness up to light and from light down again, as it always had and always will.

Field Notes

Rescue depends on an invisible infrastructure. Many of the most consequential roles in an outcome never enter the room where the decision is made.

Signal: If your system feels "held together," look for the shadow responders—dispatch, paging, transport, housekeeping, mechanics, unit clerks—quietly preventing failure.

Failure modes: Treating these roles as interchangeable, invisible, or "less clinical" degrades communication, slows response, and erodes morale that you will need during the worst night.

Practice: Learn names, learn workflows, and build reciprocal trust. When someone in the shadows makes your rescue possible, close the loop with gratitude and make that gratitude visible to their leaders.

DISCUSSION / WRITING PROMPTS (optional)

- List the "shadow roles" that contributed to your last three rescues. Add names where you can.
- Choose three shadow rescuers. Ask how they came to the role and what keeps them there. Write a short paragraph honoring each.

6 - THE WRONG SIDE OF THE SHEETS

One warm Sunday afternoon in 1983, the driver entered an intersection. He did so legally, and the eyewitness said so too. The light was green; his car began to move; and another car plowed into the driver's side—*t-boning* it, in the argot of the ambulance crew that came and whisked the driver away. The police stayed behind. They made diagrams and took statements and called a hauling company to remove the carcass of metal and glass and extruded plastic. A few hours later, the intersection had resumed its steady rhythm—cars stopping and starting and proceeding through—the crash forgotten except for a few sparkles of glass shining up from the asphalt.

That driver knew the intersection had reopened because he saw it from the back seat of a taxi taking him home from the community hospital where a kindly family physician covering the ED that morning had examined him and taken an X-ray and given him crutches and a prescription for codeine and sent him on his way, saying that the blood in his urine would clear in a few days. He hobbled into his apartment, his young wife quite concerned, and she made him chicken soup and sent him to bed.

I know this to be true, because the young wife was my wife Barbara, and the driver was me.

The next morning, I was quite stiff but reasoned that everything would be okay. I pulled on scrubs and called a taxi to take me the three miles to the other hospital where I was assigned. The taxi driver helped me stow the crutches, and when we arrived he helped me to my feet. I hobbled inside to meet the team and sat in an empty wheelchair.

The on-call intern arrived first, and then the other resident, and finally the senior resident in charge of the service. When the senior resident said it was time to start rounds, I asked the others to push me. The senior resident asked that I stop kidding around and let's get going.

"Will you help me get up?"

Only then did the senior resident notice the crutches. He wondered why I had a set of crutches, and I explained that I could not bear weight on my left hip.

In a few moments I was again on a stretcher in the back of an ambulance, this time on the way to the big hospital where I was poked and prodded. The radiologist, with blue eyes and a shock of white-blond hair, had come of professional age in the field hospitals of Vietnam. He came at me with a big syringe of contrast that made me feel boiling hot and nauseated like a cancer patient while he performed an ancient study called an intravenous pyelogram (IVP) that showed the big crack in the left kidney, and another study that showed the collection of blood around my hip joint that explained why I could not bear weight.

Some hours later, Barbara was allowed in. She had been crying.

Then my service chief came in and gently suggested that I was "a [expletive] idiot" who would have been fired for managing a patient the way I had managed myself.

He was right, of course.

I wasn't much good as a resident for the next few days. I got to count the holes in the ceiling tiles as they stared back at me. I had treatments and physical therapy and so on, and they eventually released me to get around in a wheelchair and on crutches.

The service chief came by and said I would be no good in the operating room for a while, and I was better used in the ICU where I could make rounds from a wheelchair and on crutches.

It hurt too much to go home (just across the street and a block away) so they let me sleep my off nights in the call room. Barbara made dinner and brought it over, and the other residents smelled it, and the next night she made dinner for six and it was all gone in forty-five minutes.

Ten days later I was able to go home to sleep, to eat, and to bathe, finally confident that I could make it back to the hospital when needed.

When I made it home and we finally had time to chat, Barbara did not hide her displeasure about how I had not looked after myself. I wanted nothing more than to forget the whole experience, and to do so as quickly as possible.

A Third of a Century Later

In 2019, on a winter afternoon at a conference center in San Diego, I was the penultimate speaker in the penultimate session of the meeting. I had awoken that morning feeling vaguely unwell, hoping that this was not my year to pick up the transmissible crud that surfaces any time and every time people from far distant places gather. I don't remember much about giving the talk. It was a familiar topic and a lecture I had given so many times before that the cadences and slide changes and intercalated references to Star Trek (or was it Star Wars?) came easily. But I felt warm and my mind felt fuzzy, and I chose to nap before my nurse colleague saw me waiting for a taxi to the airport. She said I looked "off" and counseled sleep during the red-eye back to Atlanta.

Sleep I did. Later, I would not recall the takeoff, or the climb, or the cruise, or the descent, or the rumble of flaps and gear or even the landing. I stumbled off the airplane just before 6 a.m. local time, and to baggage claim, and into the Uber, and finally home.

Barbara said that I looked lousy and I told her I felt lousy and I needed a nap. There was a dinner I was to host the next evening, a visiting delegation of physicians from China, and it was important—very important—that I be at my best.

The nap was more than a nap, and she had some difficulty awakening me. And then she noticed that my left leg was red. From the foot, up the calf, and coming up past my knee.

She called my doctor, who happened to be a neighbor a block away, and he made a house call (in 2019!) and looked at me and told her to take me to the hospital and not bother with the emergency room because he had already arranged for an admission and intravenous antibiotics.

I don't remember much about the admissions office. Barbara told me that I would awaken, say something unintelligible, and fall back asleep.

The redness had ascended to mid-thigh before the antibiotics forced it to retreat.

The condition is called *erysipelas*.

The cause is a bacterium called *streptococcus*.

The consequence is this thing called *sepsis*, anemically defined as "life-threatening organ dysfunction caused by the body's dysregulated response to infection, identified by an acute increase of ≥2 SOFA (Sequential Organ Failure Assessment) points."

I had an increase of 4 points—creatinine and bilirubin both elevated to 2.2 mg/dl, if you must know-- so I qualified.

Life-threatening.

Two colleagues dropped everything to host the elegant dinner for the visitors that I had invited to Atlanta. Barbara went in my place. My hospital tray held a sad turkey sandwich and a Coca-Cola product. (I am sure it was a Coca-Cola product, as other brands are neither offered nor consumed among polite Atlanta institutions.)

Some colleagues came by the next day. One of them – one who had covered my absence at the distinguished visitor dinner the prior night -- remarked that I was an internationally recognized sepsis expert and commented on the obvious irony.

Another more senior colleague came by, and upon hearing the entire story casually observed that I was "a [expletive] idiot" who would have been fired for managing a patient the way I had managed myself.

He was right, of course.

We rescuers make a sort of one-sided bargain with God, something to the effect that we will go anywhere and do anything at any time to care for the critically ill and injured.

All we ask is that we not be afflicted. It's one-sided, we know this. But we choose to overlook it, disbelieve it, and generally disregard it—until the day we wake up on the wrong side of the sheets.

That day is not a moral failure. It is a forecast.

If you live by rescue, you do not get to negotiate with biology. You do not get to outrun infection with willpower, or out-argue physiology with reputation, or buy immunity with service. You can minimize your own symptoms, white-knuckle through rounds, tell yourself you'll deal with it after the next shift—but the body keeps its own ledger. Rescue does not confer immunity. It confers exposure.

The lesson is not "be tougher."

The lesson is this: when you become the patient, stop pretending you are exempt—because the moment you notice you are "off," you are already late.

Rescuer In The Mirror

Rescuers are trained, early and often, to keep going. Attendance becomes virtue. Your own symptoms become background noise. Asking for coverage feels like weakness. It is an unexamined culture until you are the one on the wrong side of the sheets.

Dependency is its own humiliation: help me stand, I need crutches, I need a cane. The hidden gift is empathy, the embodied understanding of what our patients live with while we speak about it clinically.

Denial, however, is reflexive. We minimize, postpone, and bargain with physiology. We worry we will be seen as weak, and we forget that self-preservation is also a professional obligation.

My advice: when you notice you are "off," stop negotiating. Seek help early and let others cover you the way you would cover them. This is not surrender; it is stewardship.

Mirror question: What symptom have you been explaining away that deserves the dignity of being evaluated?

7 - HELP IS ON THE WAY

"Every rescuer stands in the light of someone who answered the call before them."

--TGB

I had been assigned to a six-month exchange rotation (January through June) as a Junior Registrar at the old Richmond Hospital in Dublin, Ireland. Barbara and I had been married two years, but she remained in Baltimore, completing her second post-doctoral fellowship. Now, midway through the rotation, I had fallen into a comfortable habit: finishing rounds, signing out to the overnight house officer, and heading to the corner pub for dinner.

One evening the senior house officer, an earnest man named Hayes, asked me to stop by casualty (the British term for the emergency department) to see a twenty-five-year-old who had stolen a car and driven it into a tree. His vital signs were stable, but he was mildly tender to gentle pressure on his abdomen.

Neither CT scan nor ultrasound was available.

Earlier that week, I demonstrated the technique of diagnostic peritoneal lavage to the junior staff: injecting local anesthetic near the umbilicus, making a tiny incision through the abdominal wall, threading in a small straw-like tube, infusing saline, and then retrieving and inspecting the fluid. I told Hayes to perform that procedure.

Fifteen minutes later, the direct hospital line rang in the pub.

"Mr. Buchman, come quickly! I've killed the patient!"

In the background, I could hear the patient asking, "What's happening to me?" Clearly, the man was very much alive. There had been a lot of blood in the abdomen, and it had shot out the moment Hayes introduced the catheter.

I trotted back to casualty, explained to the patient that we needed to take him to theatre (the operating room), and called the nurse in charge, the duty anesthetist, and the blood bank to prepare four units of blood for crossmatch.

Soon we were in theatre. The patient was anesthetized, his abdomen prepped and draped. Together, Hayes and I opened the abdomen. A suction device quickly aspirated the blood; we irrigated the remainder with saline and began searching for the source. Both lower quadrants were pristine. Suspecting the spleen, I retracted the abdominal wall so Hayes could look. "No bleeding there," he said. I looked as well. No injury.

It must be the liver, I thought. We explored under and around it. Nothing.

Hmmm.

I asked Hayes to pull hard so I could see over the dome of the liver where it met the diaphragm. There was a bit of clot, perhaps the size of a hen's egg. I swept it free.

The abdomen filled with dark venous blood at breathtaking speed. The patient's blood pressure plummeted. The anesthesiologist transfused two of the four units as I stuffed large sponges into the space between the liver and diaphragm. With pressure, the bleeding stopped.

We were in trouble. Big trouble, in fact. The injury—a laceration of the large vein running through the backside of the liver up to the heart—was described in textbooks as generally unsurvivable. I had read how to repair it, but that was book-learning. I knew I lacked both the exposure and the experience needed to save the patient.

I asked the OR sister to ring the consultant, Paul, the senior attending on call.

Paul phoned back a few minutes later. He was at a sporting event. I told him I had a patient on the table with a retrohepatic caval injury and needed help.

"If the patient is alive," he replied, "he cannot have such an injury."

Biting my tongue, swallowing my pride, I said simply, "I need you regardless."

Paul bounded in, scrubbed hands held high, quickly donning gown and gloves. He gently elbowed past Hayes. "Let's have a look." As he reached for the pile of sponges packed between the liver and diaphragm, I tried to warn him.

"Paul, go slow—"

Too late. Paul pulled the sponges free, and a tidal wave of black blood erupted. He shouted for more sponges. The anesthetist transfused the remaining two units.

"Holy Mother of God—it is a retrohepatic caval injury!" he said.

Yes, it was.

This was not a cardiac surgery hospital, but we had to find a way. Together, we reviewed the steps for exposure, control, and a shunt to temporarily redirect the blood flow—

ad hoc engineering with what we had on hand. Once more, we rehearsed the plan and began.

I carried the abdominal incision up through the chest to the base of the neck. Using the surgical equivalent of a hammer and chisel (a Lebschke knife) we split the breastbone. We opened the pericardial sac. With Hayes still holding pressure, we passed linen tape around the vena cava below the liver and again within the pericardial sac. We placed a purse-string suture in the right atrial appendage, fashioned a shunt from a plastic chest tube, inserted it into the vena cava, and cinched the linen tapes to force blood through the shunt. We clamped the portal triad to stop blood flow into the liver.

Hayes pulled away the sponges. I got the suction close. Paul, with the better angle, found the tear and quickly repaired it with polypropylene suture. We released the clamp, removed the shunt, vented the heart, and secured the purse-string.

The anesthesiologist reported that we had used eight units of blood, our entire supply.

We irrigated the chest and abdomen, placed drains to detect any recurrent bleeding, and spent the next hour closing the incisions.

Ten days later, the young man was taken to jail.

Hayes, Paul, and the entire OR team had just performed the first successful repair of a retrohepatic inferior vena caval injury in Ireland.

Rescue is a matter of preparedness, judgment, and skill—pretty much in that order.

The most successful rescuers are those who decide never to stop learning, never to stop training, never to stop improving the odds. Some are innovators, others teachers, others masters of logistics. We learn from one another.

Yet none of that mattered more in this case than one essential truth: no rescuer rescues alone.

Humility opens the door to collaboration; collaboration makes rescue possible. Survival often depends on asking for the right help at the right time and on the readiness of another rescuer to respond. Every request for assistance must be regarded as legitimate and urgent, regardless of inconvenience or cost.

The only acceptable answer is: *"I'm on my way."*

Two Decades Later

Four years had passed since the airing of "Cross Currents", my episode of Trauma: Life in the ER. Barbara and I were getting ready for bed when my pager sounded. The number belonged to the main trauma OR. When I called, the circulating nurse said that my newest hire, Dr. Douglas Schuerer, "has a situation" and needs you in the OR.

"I'm on my way."

Twenty minutes later, scrubbed hands held high, I donned gown and gloves.

"What's up?"

Doug explained that he had a patient with a gunshot wound that entered the caudate lobe of the liver. The slug appeared to have traversed the retrohepatic vena cava. Together we gently removed the sponges he had packed into the space. A tidal wave of black blood erupted. We quickly stuffed sponges back in and held pressure.

He looked at me and asked, "Didn't you save one of these in Ireland?"

We assembled the necessary tools—this time with a proper sternal saw and a more refined shunt—and went to work.

It was easier the second time. Two hours later we delivered the patient to the surgical intensive care unit. Doug and his team had achieved their first successful repair of a retrohepatic caval injury.

Two more decades have passed. I left St. Louis in 2009, having handed the leadership of the Trauma Center to Doug. He still holds that role today. And when the call comes from his young surgeons, I know how he answers.

"*I'm on my way.*"

The best rescuers never rescue alone.

Field Notes

Asking for help is not weakness; it is a clinical skill. The best teams make escalation routine and response immediate.

Signal: When you feel time pressure, uncertainty, or a sense that you are "behind the case," treat that sensation as a cue to call early.

Failure modes: The common failure is delay—"I thought I could handle it." Delay converts solvable problems into preventable disasters and isolates the rescuer.

Practice: Receive every request as legitimate. Respond with urgency and service: "Thanks for calling. I'm here. What can I do?" Give credit to the caller; they saved the patient by escalating.

DISCUSSION / WRITING PROMPTS (optional)

• When have you asked for help? How was the ask received and what did you learn from that reception?

• When have you been asked for help? How did you respond, and what would you do differently next time?

• What would you say to a colleague who should have asked for help, but didn't?

8 - A RARE AND FEARED COMPLICATION

It is the beginning of my fifth year in residency, time to choose my final path in surgery.

The new chairman of my department is a world-renowned pancreas surgeon. Though my class was chosen by his predecessor, he declares that the three of us now entering our fifth year will be his first graduating residents.

Each of us will serve a sixth year as Assistant Chief of Surgery at the Johns Hopkins Hospital before pursuing fellowship training. My two colleagues are already committed: each will mold himself in his image, become pancreas surgeons, and one day build their own academic dynasties.

I am less certain.

It is a Sunday afternoon, the last of my last rotation through the Loch Raven VA Hospital. I tell Barbara that I have a dozen charts to dictate and will be home in time for dinner. The air is warm, the sky clear, and the parking lot nearly empty. I nod to the intern covering the wards and make my way to the team office on Ward 4A.

About twenty minutes later I am somewhere in the midst of the third chart. There is a commotion in the hallway. Staff are running toward Ward 4B. That is never a good sign in any hospital, and it is an especially bad one in a VA Medical Center on a Sunday afternoon, where the intern happens to be the most senior physician on duty. I follow the noise to a room near the far end of the corridor.

The scene could have come straight from a horror film: a man wide-eyed with terror, firing a jet of blood from his neck with every beat of his heart. But this was no movie. The veteran was dying in front of us. Nurses pressed desperately, but the bleeding would not stop.

The intern gave me the story. The patient had undergone resection of an oral cancer and placement of a tracheostomy three weeks earlier to protect his airway. He had lingered in the hospital but was scheduled for discharge in the morning.

And now this.

Anatomy of a Catastrophe

The neck is a busy place. It contains the airway and the esophagus, the thyroid and parathyroid glands, and paired highways of blood vessels to and from the brain. Add the vagus nerves and lymph nodes, and it becomes a crowded neighborhood indeed.

When we perform tracheostomy, we remember the ancient caution: *There be dragons close by.*

Of the dragons, the fiercest is the brachiocephalic artery—also known, ominously, as the innominate artery, "he who will not be named." It branches from the aorta and courses just under the top of the breastbone, crossing in front of the trachea before dividing into the right common carotid and right subclavian arteries.

The tracheostomy tube passes through the front of the airway and is held in place by an inflatable balloon. We are taught to keep that balloon pressure as low as possible and the tracheostomy as high as possible so that nothing presses against the artery below.

Normally, the artery lies deep enough and well protected by fat and tissue.

Normally, but not always.

Not in a slender man.

Not in one whose tissues have been thinned by cancer, or whose tracheostomy is a bit low, or whose innominate artery rides a few centimeters higher than average. In such cases, the relentless beating of that artery against the trachea and the balloon erodes the thin wall between them. A few bacteria and their enzymes do the rest.

The result is a tracheo-innominate fistula, which is a direct connection between the airway and a major artery. It is a rare event. It is also among the most feared in all of surgery.

The textbooks offer two grim pieces of advice:

1. Be vigilant for a small "herald bleed" in the days and weeks after tracheostomy.

2. If the flood comes, the only chance of survival is to open the wound, for the surgeon to slide an index finger down alongside the trachea, and compress the artery against the breastbone.

Improvisation

The patient was long past any herald bleed. He was nearly exsanguinated, consciousness slipping away. There was no time for textbooks.

For historical reasons, house staff in our program were instructed to always carry a disposable scalpel in their uniform pocket. It was my day off. I had none that Sunday afternoon.

The intern, mercifully, did.

I pulled on gloves and asked for his scalpel. There was neither time nor need for local anesthesia, because the man was moments from death. I made the incision, slid my finger down alongside the trachea, pressed forward, and said a silent prayer.

The bleeding stopped.

The heart beat on.

Proof of life.

A respiratory therapist connected an AMBU bag to force oxygen into the patient's lungs. I told the surgical intern to find a vein at the ankle, insert the largest IV he could, and start infusing saline. The medical intern arrived, and I sent her to the blood bank: "Bring whatever compatible blood they have. If you have to, call the director. Just get it here."

The nurse supervisor, the most senior nurse in the hospital that afternoon. appeared at the doorway. I told her we needed to move to the operating room. She reminded me what we both already knew: the OR was locked, and the on-call anesthesiologist was forty-five minutes away.

"Call security," I said. "Get it unlocked. Call my attending and the anesthesiologist. Tell them to get here as fast as they can."

The patient opened his eyes. My index finger was still inside his chest, holding the pressure point that kept him alive.

"We've got the bleeding under control," I told him quietly, "but we have to go to the operating room to fix the problem." He nodded faintly and squeezed the nurse's hand.

The medical intern returned with two units of low-titer type O blood—universal donor. "I didn't wait for the crossmatch," she said.

"Right call," I told her. She squeezed the blood through the tubing by hand.

His color improved. His blood pressure steadied. It was time to move.

The challenge: my finger could not move from the artery.

"Slide him to the far left side of the bed," I said. They did. And then I climbed up beside him.

We rode together supine to the operating room—he and I, side by side—my index finger keeping him alive.

Another Improvisation

Neither my attending nor the anesthesiologist had yet arrived. The nurse supervisor looked at me, anxious.

Five years earlier, as a senior medical student, I had spent a month on elective with an anesthesiologist, curious about their work. That curiosity now paid an unexpected dividend.

"Roll the anesthesia machine over here," I told the intern. "Flip those two switches, set the tidal volume to seven hundred milliliters, end-expiratory pressure to five." From the fog of time long past with an anesthesiologist who insisted I learn, a mantra returned: *Three of the blue, two of the green, and one of some other colored gas*. "Turn those knobs-three liters per minute of nitrous oxide, two of oxygen, and one percent of whatever's in the vaporizer."

We connected the tubing to the tracheostomy. Within a minute, the patient drifted to sleep.

Just then, my surgery attending arrived. He had never seen this complication either, but we both had read the books and knew what had to be done: widen the incision, find the artery, clamp it, and if necessary, split the upper breastbone.

Moments later the anesthesiologist appeared. He was understandably unhappy that his machine and gases had been conscripted. The surgery attending intervened. "Let's save the patient first," he said, "and discuss it later."

The anesthesiologist intubated through the mouth with elegant speed. We enlarged the incision around my finger, retracted the tissues, and at last saw the torn artery. The only chance was to tie it off. We got proximal and distal control, ligated it, and waited. The bleeding stopped once more, this time for good.

Aftermath

For the next week, a nurse was stationed at the bedside to change the gauze on the open wound every thirty minutes until the tracheal defect had sealed. The patient recovered fully—awake, intact, and astonishingly without neurological deficit.

The anesthesiologist had pulled me aside. His tone was stern but his eyes not unkind. "Don't ever touch my machine again," he said. Then, after a pause: "How did you know what to do?"

I told him the name of the man who had drilled the basics of anesthetics into me during my student years.

He grinned. "I know that guy."

I made it home in time for dinner, with a story to tell Barbara.

The patient made it out of the hospital alive.

Months later, I was summoned to the chairman's office. He asked about my career plans. "Trauma, emergency surgery, and critical care," I told him.

He expressed dismay. In his view, such a path was unworthy of a Hopkins super chief. It was not the way to build an empire.

But I had already learned, on a quiet Sunday afternoon at the Loch Raven VA, that rescue—not empire—was the work that mattered to me most.

Rescuer In The Mirror

High-stakes rescues are never scheduled. Familiar crises can be drilled and choreographed; catastrophes cannot. They arrive fast, short on people and knowledge and time.

A catastrophe cannot be allowed to become chaos. Someone must impose cadence, break the work into familiar tasks, and assign roles to the best available hands. Speed is fine; accuracy is final.

Improvisation is not freelancing. It is disciplined adaptation: raise concerns once, clearly; acknowledge alternatives; then execute the simplest plan that can work. Leaders must be self-aware, because their affect becomes the room's physiology.

My advice: after the save, stay open to the debrief. Praise and complaint can arrive together. Listen, extract the lesson, give credit widely, and remember that the remembered thing will be the grace of the save—not your ownership of it.

Mirror question: In a true catastrophe, what is your first move? Control the room? Or control yourself?

9 - LEARNING TO ASK, ASKING TO LEARN

The VA experience had taught me that sometimes rescue demands improvisation—the courage to act when no script exists.

But not every rescue is born of audacity. Some come quietly, from humility, curiosity, and the willingness to ask. If the prior lesson was about the power of doing, this one was about the power of learning, especially learning from those who knew what I did not yet know.

I had completed the Assistant Chief of Service ("Super Chief") year at Hopkins. It had been an unforgettable crucible of growth. After some interesting negotiation, my chairman, the one initially dismayed with my choice, decided that it was finally time to establish a faculty-led Adult Trauma Service at Hopkins, adjacent to the time-honored Halsted Service run by the Assistant Chiefs. He gave me a go-ahead, the closest thing to his blessing.

Part of the agreement involved a year across town at the Maryland Institute for Emergency Medical Services Systems—MIEMSS, or as everyone else called it, Shock Trauma. The state-run institute received the lion's share of Maryland's serious injuries, and I reasoned that whatever protocols and procedures they had developed there could serve as a foundation for building the Hopkins service.

The problem was simple: I didn't know what I didn't know. And I didn't yet know how—or from whom—I would learn.

A Night to Remember

One evening is etched in memory. I was rotating through the Critical Care Resuscitation Unit—Shock Trauma's version of an ICU—caring for a young man who had chosen not to wear a seatbelt. In a contest between an irresistible force (a car moving at fifty miles an hour) and an immovable object (a large oak tree), the car lost. He was ejected and badly injured. Among the casualties were his lungs.

We rescuers tend to keep things simple: the air goes in and out, and the blood goes round and round. Everything else is details.

When the lungs are damaged, oxygen can't pass efficiently into the bloodstream. We worry about that so much that we put red lights on patients 'fingers to measure oxygen levels—those pulse oximeters that translate light absorption into a number on the monitor. You and I, assuming we're healthy, run about 97–99%. That's the percentage of hemoglobin molecules carrying oxygen.

When the percent saturation drops into the low 90s, we administer oxygen. If it falls again, we place a breathing tube and start a mechanical ventilator.

The ventilator was brand new, bristling with switches and dials. One controlled the percent of oxygen delivered.

We breathe 21% oxygen in room air; the ventilator could deliver up to 100%. Other controls adjusted the pressure and the volume of each breath. The goal: keep that saturation number high enough to sustain life.

My patient had been intubated on arrival. As I passed his bed, I saw the oxygen level -the percent saturation-had slipped from 97 down to 92. It was time to act.

I increased the oxygen concentration. The number rose briefly to 95, then started to fall again. I turned it up higher. No response. Now 87. At 87% oxygen saturation, the room gets quieter. Everyone knows what that number means.

I turned the dial so the patient was receiving pure oxygen. The lungs laughed. The oxygen saturation percent in the arteries dropped again—to 85.

I ordered an emergency chest X-ray. The film, which should have shown black air-filled lungs, instead showed a blizzard of white.

I began increasing the ventilator pressures. The oxygen saturation percent was now 80—then 77. That's a "if we don't turn this around, he'll be dead within the hour" situation.

I was out of magic.

The Call

In 1987, attending physicians on call carried pagers—and quarters for the pay phone. (If you're under thirty and have no idea what "quarters and a pay phone" mean, ask someone who remembers the last century.)

Except for one attending: Howard.

Howard was a fireplug of a man with curly hair and a scruffy beard, a tech nerd before the word existed. He had queued up to buy one of the first IBM PCs six years earlier and, more impressively, had also bought a Motorola DynaTAC mobile telephone. (Again, ask someone who remembers the last century, or just Google it.)

His number was scrawled on an index card taped to the nurses' station. I called him. He answered from a baseball game at the old Memorial Stadium. I told him the situation.

He flagged down a police officer, flashed his ShockTrauma credentials, and was at the bedside in ten minutes.

"Glad you called," he said, calm as ever.

He ambled over to the ventilator and began turning dials. Thirty seconds later, the oxygen level stopped falling. A minute later, it was rising. Within five minutes, it was 100%. The patient's blood was fully saturated with oxygen.

The nurses and I just stared.

Howard smiled, nodded once, and went back to the ballgame.

Three Questions

After morning rounds, I found him and asked three questions.

First: "What did you do?"

Second: "How did you know what to do?"

It was the ventilator, he explained. The vent was a new model with a mode designed precisely for this kind of lung injury. (For the medical readers: the vent was a Siemens Servo 900C, and the mode was pressure-controlled inverse ratio ventilation, newly described at the time.)

He picked up a piece of chalk and drew on the blackboard, sketching the pressure waveforms and explaining how alveoli (the tiny air sacs) needed to be "popped open" and held open long enough for oxygen to diffuse across into the blood. I peppered him with questions, and he answered until I understood.

Coda

In the decades that followed, I would pick up color markers and go to whiteboards and channel my inner Howard, teaching generations of fellows when and why and how to use this mode of ventilation. And each time, I retold the story of that summer evening: how Howard worked his magic, saved a life, and taught a fellow who would pass the lesson forward.

And every year, without fail, a student would inquire, "So, what was the third question you asked him?"

I always paused before answering.

"Howard," I had asked, "who won the ball game?"

He grinned. "The Orioles!"

Requiem

Howard died in 2023. But he's still with us in every one of his fellows, and in every bedside lesson about how to save a life by asking the right question.

Because sometimes, learning to ask is how we learn to rescue.

Rescuer In The Mirror

Uncertainty is the native climate of rescue, and its danger is that it feels normal. The first skill is not certainty; it is noticing the gap—the patient is drifting, the story does not fit, or your plan is no longer working.

Once you see the gap, escalation becomes technique. Knowing who to call and how to reach them is not politeness; it is clinical infrastructure. Test communications early, normalize consultation, and treat the call as a deliberate intervention.

My advice: call sooner than your pride prefers. When someone helps, close the loop with gratitude because gratitude strengthens the network you will need again. In time, you will be the one who is called. Answer the way you hope others answered you.

Mirror question: What keeps you from making the call—scarcity, pride, or fear of being seen as uncertain?

10 - VERY BADLY BURNED

Firefighters command special respect from me.

Not because they rush into burning buildings. They do. Not because they are in constant danger of toxic fumes, superheated gases, and structural collapse. They are. And not because they maintain their quarters and cook for themselves. That is part of the job.

They command my special respect because they are the first responders to some of the most complex patients to ever cross my stretcher: the patient with total body full-thickness burns.

Let me assure you: the skin is a vital organ. Larger than the heart or liver or lungs, an adult's skin is massive—perhaps twenty to twenty-five square feet and eight pounds. It has essential functions: regulating heat loss, sweating, and housing the most complex set of sensory end-organs anywhere in the body. There are mechanoreceptors and nociceptors and thermoreceptors and hair-follicle receptors. There are systems to heal breaks, systems to keep water out, systems to slough dead cells and replace living ones. Some skin is exquisitely thin (like that of the eyelids); some is thick and tough (such as the skin of the back).

It all has to work. Even if you have a paper cut. Even if you have a sunburn. Even if you have a scald that blisters. The skin has to heal and regenerate and make you whole.

This is why full-thickness burns are terrifying. The skin is gone. The mechanisms that protect you are gone. The sensation is gone. The capacity for healing and regrowth is gone. In its place is dead tissue, which is a perfect culture medium.

This is why burn surgeons long ago gravitated toward early excision and grafting for smaller full-thickness wounds. They remove the dead stuff. They cover what remains with split-thickness grafts. Those grafts are never as strong or as durable as what was burned and cut away, but at least the rot is gone. At least the body is given something it can live with.

There is an old (yet still fairly reliable) rule-of-thumb estimator of mortality in full-thickness burns: age in years plus the percent of the body burned full thickness. Burn care has gotten better and the survival odds have gotten better, especially with smaller wounds in younger and healthier patients. For mid-sized burns, there has been welcome progress.

Still, age plus percent full-thickness burn gives a first estimate of mortality. And even when that number exceeds 100, we all still try to save that life.

But there is a hard truth, harder to say out loud: it doesn't matter how fast the victim is transported to a burn center. It doesn't matter the skill of the surgeon or the brilliance of the team. A really big bad burn where age plus percent full thickness burn exceeds 100 is almost certainly unsurvivable.

The firefighters know this.

Still, they try to rescue.

Still, they bring these patients to the burn center.

Still, they and we try, even when we know the outcome.

There is often a transient blessing: full-thickness burns destroy the skin's pain sensors. These patients sometimes need far less pain medication than anticipated. Often, they are lucid.

For a while.

Then the skin becomes leathery and inelastic, and in order to let them breathe we sometimes have to cut a checkerboard into the charred black leather of their chest and sides and back. This is called escharotomy. The burn victims feel no pain when we split the char because their pain sensors no longer exist.

But the rest of the organs know. The body knows.

The kidneys stop making urine. The liver falters, unable to metabolize nutrients or make clotting factors. The gut forgets how to absorb. The immune system, stripped of its first and best line of defense, is forced into a sudden and terrible war.

It is only a matter of time.

In the cryptic language of triage, the patient is color-coded the same as their newly charred skin: black. There is a gentle euphemism for management priority: expectant. Let me translate that.

We moisten whatever lips are unburned. We give morphine in abundance to ease whatever pain remains (it is usually not much). And we rush to find the next of kin.

Time is not on their side. They may have minutes. Perhaps an hour or two if they were young and healthy before the catastrophe.

The real goal of our care is brutally simple: find a way to let them say *I love you.*

I will always love you.

Goodbye.

These are the hardest words for the victim, harder still for their loved ones.

They are also hard for we rescuers.

Sometimes there is a plaintive wail: isn't there something, anything, to give us a few more minutes… an hour… a day?

There is not.

We are left to bear witness to a tragedy that was inconceivable a few hours ago, one that now none of us can avert. Not the firefighter, nor the paramedic, nor the EMT, nor the policeman, nor the ED nurse, nor the burn surgeon. Each has done everything to effect rescue. But it is not enough to save this life.

The vital organs no longer work. The harmonies of their interactions are silenced. The wisdom of the body fades to nothing. The victim takes their last breath. The heart stops. A crisp white sheet is laid across them.
Someone looks at the clock and announces the time.

Firefighters command my special respect because they do not turn away from this. They bring the patient anyway. They carry the weight of what they already know, and they keep their hands steady. They watch. They pray.

And when the room goes quiet—when the monitor is switched off and the sheet is drawn—something else becomes visible. Not failure. Not incompetence. Just the limits of what human beings can do for each other, and the tenderness of what we still try to do anyway.

Often the last sound in the room is a loved one speaking the same words again and again, as if repetition could hold the world in place: *I love you.*

I will always love you.

There are rescues we measure in lives saved.

And there are harder rescues that consist of a few final minutes, protected from chaos, in which love is spoken aloud and received.

The firefighters come for both.

Rescuer In The Mirror

There are rescues where skill can change the endpoint, and rescues where skill can only soften the suffering. Extensive burns are often the latter: prolonged, intimate, and relentless in every sensory dimension.

When death is not fast, the rescuer's attention becomes a kind of exposure. We focus outward so intensely that the inward questions arrive later. What could I have done? Did I do enough? Those questions linger like the smell of that char that does not ever wash fully away..

My advice: name the reality early. Sometimes rescue begins and ends with bearing witness, reducing pain, and protecting dignity. When you carry those cases home, do not carry them alone: use your team, your rituals, and your counseling resources before the dreams start writing their own field notes.

Mirror question: When rescue cannot save a life, what does "doing your job well" mean to you?

11 - INFORMED CONSENT

If I accept the sunshine and warmth, then I must also accept the thunder and lightning.

-a paraphrase of Khalil Gibran (The Prophet)

The making of a surgeon begins with training. It never ends. There are, however, milestones along the path: the first incision; the first time you are entrusted to operate alone; the final oral examination and the privilege of being called board-certified; the first day you are fully credentialed as an attending surgeon; the first business card. (Mine read: General, Thoracic, and Vascular Surgery.)

There is one other milestone, seldom named and never celebrated: the first time a patient walks in under their own power, you operate, and things go sideways. The first time a patient wakes paralyzed. The first time the patient dies.

Every surgeon reaches that milestone.

This is how I reached mine.

He was a slender man, perhaps five-foot-eight and one hundred and fifty pounds wet, with sandy hair and an easy smile. He had a wife and two sons. He had just turned fifty-seven when he came to see me at the old Baltimore City Hospital.

Like so many men from that part of the city, he was a hard smoker. His thumb and first two fingers were perpetually brown from the unfiltered cigarettes that kept him awake while he drove a tractor-trailer up and down the Eastern Seaboard. I learned later that his loads supplied the produce shelves of the Giant supermarket where Barbara shopped for our dinner. He had nourished us, however indirectly.

Two years earlier he had developed chest pain. The workup revealed blocked coronary arteries, and the heart surgeons performed the expected miracle: they rerouted blood to starving myocardium, and he survived. He went back to the road, back to delivering lettuce and tomatoes and whatever else would later end up in our kitchen.

But his troubles did not end with his sternotomy scar. His vision began to falter, briefly and strangely, as if a shade had been drawn and released. A cascade of tests led to a diagnosis with an innocent sound: carotid stenosis.

His left carotid artery - the vessel that supplies blood to the left side of the brain, the part that makes understanding and speech possible and powers the right side of the body – that conduit had narrowed. Its lining had become shaggy, much like the arteries in his heart. In his own words, he needed to be "roto-rootered" so he could keep driving the truck that delivered fresh produce to the store where Barbara bought our groceries so we could have dinner.

The operation is called carotid endarterectomy: a gentle name for a delicate procedure. It begins with a general anesthetic and an incision along the anterior border of the sternocleidomastoid muscle. The dissection passes through the platysma and into the deeper planes until the carotid sheath comes into view.

Inside that sheath lie the jugular vein, the vagus nerve, and the object of our search: the common carotid artery. The artery must be freed from surrounding tissues and controlled so blood can be temporarily halted. The dissection continues cephalad toward the angle of the jaw until the two main branches - the internal carotid and the external carotid - can be separately controlled.

Then the operation begins in earnest. The artery is opened, and decades of fat, calcium, and fibrous debris are teased out in a single, careful plane. "Roto-rootered," as promised. The hard part is up high, just as the artery passes behind the angle of the jaw towards its destination inside the skull: disease does not stop neatly, but exposure does. The jaw can only be lifted so far. At the top, the plaque must be feathered into a smooth ramp so blood does not feel invited to clot.

All in all, carotid endarterectomy is usually a rewarding procedure for both patient and surgeon.

Usually.

Every operation carries risk. Part of surgery is the continuing practice of informed consent: a responsible surgeon explains why a procedure is proposed, what benefit is expected, what risks accompany it, and what alternatives exist. He wanted to keep driving, and the procedure should reduce the risk of stroke and relieve the warning symptoms that had brought him to me.

Then came the recitation. Bleeding. Infection. Drainage. Nerve injury. And the outcomes we name with care because they are the ones that matter most: stroke and death. Less than five percent, I said, and at the time that sounded small to both of us.

As for alternatives, we could continue with anticoagulation. But that meant weekly blood draws, constant monitoring, and the inconvenience of managing a fragile medication while he lived on the road, moving food from field to shelf.

He signed the paper. I performed the operation exactly as I said I would. He woke up speaking and moving and joking in the recovery room. When I saw him before I went home that night, his wife and two sons were at the bedside, smiling. Everyone was relieved. Everyone was grateful. Everyone believed the danger had passed.

My phone rang around five in the morning.

A resident was on the line. Behind her voice I could hear shouting - the alarmed urgency of a unit that had abruptly turned toward crisis. My patient could not speak. He could not move the right side of his body. The part powered by the left brain - the part supplied by the artery I had operated on - had gone silent.

That "less than five percent" risk, which had sounded like a distant abstraction, was now one hundred percent.

"Call the operating room. Get him up there. I will meet you."

She did. I did. Within minutes we had the artery isolated and reopened. We removed clot. We restored flow.

But we were too late. Something had happened in the middle of the night while he slept, and while I slept. A portion of his brain had died.

I came out of the operating room and took his wife and sons into the small room reserved for just such occasions. I sat down with them and told them what had happened. I told them it was a serious complication. I told them I did not yet know how it would end. I told them I would care for him as best I knew how.

No, he would not be going home tomorrow. Not the next day, either.

He never moved his right side again. He never spoke again. He left the hospital in a wheelchair, went to rehabilitation, returned with sores and infections that come when a body cannot reposition itself, and eventually he died.

I presented him twice at Morbidity and Mortality conference.

The first time was when he left for rehab. I stood at the lectern and recited his history, displayed the imaging, and described the operation as routine because it had been. There were no unexpected events until the phone call and the second operation. The discussion was brief. I had done right by taking him back to the operating room, they said. This happens sometimes. And then they moved on to the next case.

I presented him again when he returned and, despite everything we did, the pneumonias and ulcers and infections of immobility overwhelmed what was left of his body and he died. I stood at the lectern once more and recapitulated the past and told the present. My words hung in the air. No one spoke. And then they moved on to the next case.

Later that day, an older surgeon - one who had crossed these milestones before I was born - came to my office. He closed the door and sat down.

"There's only one surefire way to avoid deaths and complications," he began.

He had my full and undivided attention.

"You have to give up surgery to do so."

The silence was deafening.

He went on. "This might be your first, but it will not be the last time you hurt a patient. There will be others."

I asked him how he dealt with it. He looked past me, out the window, somewhere far away.

"You don't 'deal' with it. Those cases become part of you. They remind you that we are humans caring for other humans, and sometimes things go wrong."

Then he said the sentence I still carry: "Consent is not just permission to cut on another human being. It's an acknowledgement - you and the patient together - that sometimes things go wrong."

After he left, I sat alone for a few minutes before heading down to clinic to meet the next patient sent to me for surgical care.

I spent a quarter-century as an operating surgeon before transitioning full-time into critical care medicine. I have not picked up a scalpel in an operating room for more than a decade and a half. Barbara and I have moved across the country twice since I stood at that lectern.

But there are still supermarkets. Trucks still pull up and unload produce so that Barbara can shop for our salad for the evening. And sometimes, without warning, my mind returns to a sandy-haired driver with tobacco-stained hands who came to me so he could keep doing his work – and taught me what it would take for me to continue to do mine.

Rescuer In The Mirror

In training, we learn to speak of risk in percentages, as if numbers could keep tragedy at a distance. "Less than five percent" sounds small until it becomes a phone call at five in the morning, and the percentage becomes a person. In that moment, a second patient arrives who will never appear in the chart: the rescuer who must keep functioning while carrying what happened.

This is the hard truth of procedural work: no matter how disciplined you are, no matter how competent, no matter how well-intentioned, the odds eventually catch up. If you operate long enough, you will hurt someone. You hurt them not because you were careless, but because biology is not a contract and night does not pause for your fatigue. The complication you explained honestly will someday come home to you.

That is why informed consent is more than a signature or a speech. It is a shared acknowledgment of reality. It is also a forecast of what the work will demand of the clinician when the risk becomes real. The patient and family live the consequences in the body. The clinician lives them in the mind: replaying the steps, interrogating each choice, searching for the moment that might have bent the outcome. Some of that scrutiny is necessary; it is how we improve. But some of it is a trap: the fantasy that perfect competence guarantees safety, and that a bad outcome therefore proves moral failure.

The older surgeon's counsel is both mercy and warning: those cases become part of you. You do not "get over" them. You absorb them. They change how you consent. They change how you sleep. They change how you meet the next person who is about to trust you with their body.

My advice: prepare for the second victim before you become one. Speak risk plainly, and also build a plan for the aftermath. Who you will call, how you will debrief, where you will tell the unvarnished truth, and how you will accept support without converting it into defensiveness? When the complication happens (as it inevitably will) do not disappear. Stay accountable to the patient and family, and let a trusted colleague stand beside you so you are not forced to carry the aftermath alone.

Mirror question: When the odds finally catch you, will you turn the pain into secrecy and self-punishment—or into honesty, learning, and the resolve to keep caring without hardening?

12 - NOT NOW, NOT TODAY

I returned to Johns Hopkins following my fellowship across town at Shock Trauma. My first assignment was to develop a faculty-led Adult Trauma Service, eventually absorbing the trauma activity from the resident-run Halsted Service. I anticipated a five-to-seven-year transition, a transition long enough for the new interns to mature into Halsted Super Chiefs who had never known a time when the faculty-led Adult Trauma Service didn't exist.

That fall, I passed my Board examinations in General Surgery and also the newly created Board exam in Surgical Critical Care. (It was the first year it was offered. I was awarded certificate #40.) For the next seven years, every Friday from 7 a.m. until 7 a.m. Saturday, I lived in the hospital, each case a chance to teach an intern and a third-year resident the principles and practice of trauma care.

The Reluctant Appointment

A few months later, I was summoned to the Chairman's office. An accreditation site visit loomed, and one of the requirements was a designated Surgical ICU Director. Since I was the only faculty member whose fellowship had included ICU training and culminated in board certification, he announced that I would fill that role. He was distressed when I initially declined.

I explained that the same regulation required not only a director but also dedicated housestaff (of which there were none.) He countered that he could spare at most one resident for part of the year. I made a counteroffer: I would accept the appointment as co-Director, provided the Chairman of Anesthesiology did the same and supplied housestaff. We would run the SICU as a joint enterprise between the two departments.

My Chairman was understandably circumspect about my proposal to "give away half of the SICU," but we had no alternative that would satisfy accreditation. And so, I became co-Director of the Surgical Intensive Care Unit. That role brought unexpected joy. I re-encountered the nurses who had watched me evolve from a frightened junior house officer to an overconfident senior, and finally to an attending trauma surgeon. We had become a professional family. They doted on our young daughter, who visited occasionally while Barbara worked in her lab one building over. Months became seasons; seasons became years.

Alpha Trauma

One Friday night, the pager blared:

"Alpha Trauma Team to the ED, Alpha Trauma Team to the ED."

"Alpha" was the highest level of alert, indicating that a critical patient was inbound and attending surgeon response was required immediately.

I hurried down the stairs, through the basement corridor, and entered the trauma bay just as the crew rolled in the stretcher.

"Female, about 30, pregnant. High-speed motor vehicle collision. She hit the steering wheel hard."

"Looks like a bad pelvic fracture. Pressure 70 palp, pulse 120."

She was in shock. Orthopaedics and Obstetrics were needed. I shouted for the clerk to page them stat. Two large IVs, warmed fluids, and Type O negative blood, a universal donor that was appropriate for a woman of childbearing age. Quick films: cervical spine, chest, pelvis.

The obstetrician could find no fetal heart tones. The pelvis film suggested rupture of the uterus; the bone itself was fractured from impact.

"We're pumping blood. Her pressure is 80."

We planned for massive transfusion during pelvic stabilization, followed by abdominal exploration to control internal bleeding. Registration had listed her as Jane Doe. Then, someone found an ID badge among the cut-away clothing and called out her name.

Jane Doe was one of my SICU nurses.

The Operation

We raced to the OR. She was moved to the table, painted from neck to knees with brown antiseptic. Drapes flew into place. The anesthesiologist ran saline through one IV and blood through the other, administering medication to erase pain and memory. He nodded. "Go."

The orthopedic surgeon drilled pins into each iliac crest and connected them with steel rod, thus building a bridge to close the pelvis and slow the bleeding. Then it was our turn. The obstetric resident and I opened the abdomen. Blood poured forth. A segment of bowel was torn.

The uterus had ruptured. The unborn child had taken the full force of impact. That image is burned forever into memory, but there was no time to mourn. We tied off bleeders, resected and repaired bowel, and re-approximated what remained of the uterus. Whether it would ever bear life again, we could not know. We washed, closed, and brought her to the SICU.

Family in Scrubs

Every professional who works in the ICU has honed words to comfort terrified families. That night, we spoke those soothing scripts to each other. The SICU nurses now had to care for one of their own. They rose magnificently, trading shifts when emotions ran too close to the surface, maintaining the same exacting standards they provided every other patient.

Together, we shepherded her through a bout of pneumonia and bloodstream infection. Day by day, she improved. Three weeks later, she was ready for transfer to the ward. Bowel function had returned; her color was back; physical therapy was mobilizing her daily.

During morning rounds, as we reviewed another patient's chart, a shout split the air:

"Crash cart to Room 4! I need the doctor now!"

She had stopped speaking, turned blue, and was pulseless. No time to think. Two nurses rolled her, sliding a backboard beneath her. Another began compressions.

I took the head of the bed, removed the headboard, sealed the mask over her face, and squeezed the AMBU bag.

There was still an ECG tracing but we detected no pulse. We cycled compressors, pushed epinephrine and calcium, and ruled out tension pneumothorax. Still no pulse. Prayers—spoken and silent—filled the room. We squared off against the Reaper.

Not now, Reaper. Not today.

The next compressor stepped back; I reached again for her neck.

"I have a pulse. Check the radial."

"Pulse at the wrist."

Not now, Reaper. Not today.

She survived the crash, the infection, and the cardiac arrest. She made it to rehab. A year later, she appeared in my clinic. All the metabolic chaos had left her with gallstones, and her internist recommended cholecystectomy.

I offered a referral to one of our expert gallbladder surgeons.

She shook her head.

"If I'd wanted one of them, I'd be in their clinic. No one is going inside my abdomen except you."

I couldn't persuade her otherwise.

The next week, I removed her gallbladder. She sailed through surgery. She never returned to service in the SICU—none of us would have, given those memories.

We all remembered her rescue as equal parts triumph and terror. Then, one day, news reached us that gave the unit reason to celebrate: The uterine repair had held. She had given birth to a healthy baby.

Rescuer In The Mirror

Some days we do hand-to-hand combat with death. When we win, it is almost never because of one person. It is because a team converges with timing, skill, and a shared refusal.

The danger after a win is the story we tell ourselves, a story that we have pushed death away for good. We have not. Even survival can carry syndromes of fear, dependence, and the long rehabilitation of trust in one's own body.

My advice: celebrate briefly, then stay honest about the downstream. Winning is rarely a return to baseline; it is a new life with new constraints. Walk with patients and families long enough to see what your "save" became—and let that knowledge mature your definition of success.

Mirror question: What kind of win are you chasing? An arrest reversed? Or a life made livable afterward?

13 - CROSSBOW

On a June afternoon in 1987, a woman named Jewel who was deep into her last trimester walked toward her modest home in a rundown section of Baltimore. The day was unseasonably warm, and the heat had pulled people onto their stoops. Most were simply sitting, watching the street, letting the hours pass.

Two men were not content to sit.

A disagreement turned into a shouting match. Tempers rose faster than the temperature. One of the men stormed inside and came back with a hunter's crossbow. He raised it, aimed quickly, and pulled the trigger. The bolt leapt forward, clearing the railing in a split second.

A few dozen yards away, Jewel took what would be her last step.

The bolt entered low, under the ribcage, punched through the diaphragm, and kept going through the unglamorous, essential anatomy of the upper abdomen. There was nothing theatrical about it. It was physics and soft tissue, speed and luck, and then the sudden calculus of blood that should have returned to her heart spilling out.

There was a lot of blood.

The ambulance arrived. The crew loaded her, secured her, flipped on the lights and siren, and drove the ten blocks to the trauma center.

We waited, each of us gloved and gowned in thin disposable fabric. We stood arrayed around the bay with the practiced stillness of a team poised at the edge of urgency. I was leading.

They rolled her in.

There was a lot of blood.

She had neither pulse nor pressure. I took a scalpel, opened her chest, clamped the aorta, and began cardiac massage with my hands. I squeezed her motionless heart, compressing it directly while others pushed saline and whatever fluid they could scrounge into her veins.

Then I told someone else to squeeze.

I had noticed what everyone had noticed but no one had said out loud: she was near term. And I also knew what I had just done. The moment I clamped the aorta, I redirected what little blood flow might have remained away from her lower body, away from her uterus, away from the baby.

I picked up the scalpel again. I opened her abdomen, found the uterus, incised it, and delivered her baby. Such a cesarean section (C-section) was the way my father (an OB/GYN) had brought so many babies into the world.

There was a lot of blood.

Her baby did not breathe. The neonatologists whisked the infant away and did what neonatologists sometimes do: they pulled life back from the narrowest ledge.

Jewel's heart never beat again. Her baby's heart did beat, but only for a day.

They were buried together.

I had a wife. We had a new baby at home. I could not imagine either without the other. I could not imagine them without me.

Two days later, the phone rang.

Jewel carried the AIDS virus.

There had been a lot of blood. And we had been covered in it.

For the next three months, I lived in a peculiar borderland. I was uncertain whom to tell, uncertain what to do, uncertain who I would be if the answer went the other way.

I had my blood drawn far from the hospital where I worked. It was my right, my attorney said: my right to know, and my right not to disclose even if a test came back positive. As long as I didn't bleed on someone else, it was my right to remain a rescuer.

Was that the same as the right to remain a husband? A father?

More to the point, I was scared. Back then, there was no treatment for HIV. My wife was scared too: scared for me, scared for herself, and scared for our infant daughter.

At one month, I tested negative. Again at two months. Again at three months.

I was clear. I was clean. I could go back to being a rescuer, a husband, a father.

Jewel and her child stayed with me. They visit my dreams from time to time, reminding me that rescuers are not invulnerable. We are vulnerable to the memories of the rescue that fails. We are vulnerable to the dispassionate ambition of microbes to spread. We are no less vulnerable than those we try to rescue.

Sometimes that June afternoon returns without warning. A fragment surfaces unbidden, and with the insistence of something unfinished.

I recall this one thing above all else.

There was a lot of blood.

Rescuer In The Mirror

Rescues unfold in real time. Training, protocols, people, consumables, and transport converge, and we act inside the seconds we are given. When outcomes are clean, either simple success or rapid failure, the emotional physics dissipate quickly.

The hard cases are the ones that do not resolve. A dramatic save can leave a long tail: fears about exposure, questions about judgment, and the unsettling awareness that a single case can ripple through marriage, parenthood, and identity.

My advice: take care of your home system with the same seriousness you take care of your patients. The bargain of rescue does not include immunity, and it does not guarantee that someone will always rescue you in return. Hold your people close, and do not postpone the conversations that matter.

Mirror question: What case are you still carrying as unfinished? What would "closure" realistically look like?

14 - THE NEXT GENERATION

Our episode of Trauma: Life in the ER ("Cross Currents") aired on Tuesday, November 2, 1999. The hospital hosted a watch party, and I took my share of gentle ribbing. I hadn't realized how popular the show was until a few weeks later, while boarding an airport shuttle in Philadelphia. As I handed the driver my luggage, he squinted at me and remarked that I looked like "a TV doctor."

I was looking forward to the holidays. People grew kinder, the tide of violence ebbed, the elective OR schedule thinned, and a vague peace settled over both the hospital and the city.

Eighteen months later, around the time that summer was yielding to fall, I was finishing paperwork when my secretary, Gloria, appeared in the doorway.

"What's up?"

"There's a call for you on line 1," she said, pausing. "I think you should say yes."

Gloria settled into the chair opposite me. She was clearly intending to listen in. I hit the speakerphone.

"Hello, Tim Buchman here."

A tiny voice replied, "Hello, my name is Penelope. I saw the TV show. I want to come shadow you. It's for a school project."

I scribbled a note and held it up to Gloria: What grade is she in?

Gloria flashed nine fingers.

"Penelope, thanks for calling. Is your mom around? Can she join us on the phone?"

Penelope's mother picked up a few seconds later. I gently explained that the trauma service was a stressful place, a place where people came in shot, stabbed, or broken from car wrecks. Some weren't people you'd invite home for dinner.

Sometimes they died.

Her mother didn't flinch. "Penelope has seen the shows. Since she saw your episode, it's all she talks about. She has a school project to complete. If you won't do this, we'll call your colleague across town and see if he will."

Gloria crossed her arms, eyebrow raised. She gave the universal "mom look" that meant *Don't you dare disappoint this child.*

We compromised on a three-hour evening visit: her parents would drop her off, have dinner, and return later.

I silently prayed to the trauma gods for peace during that interval.

First Visit

The appointed evening arrived. I briefed the medical student, intern, and resident that we'd have a high school freshman shadowing. We met Penelope and her parents by the lobby fountain. The team was instantly charmed. Someone found her a pair of XXS scrubs (the smallest size available) and off we went to the Emergency Department.

I stepped aside for a phone call. When I returned, Penelope was being shown around by the charge nurse. Our young visitor toured the trauma bay, sat at the CT scanner console where the TV crew had filmed, watched a laceration repair, and observed a cast being applied. She asked sharp, curious questions, and the staff answered with easy kindness.

We continued to the operating rooms, which were quiet that night. The circulating and scrub nurses decided she should not only see an OR, but also learn to scrub. In a few moments she was fully dressed with cap, mask, gown, and gloves.

There were no smartphones in those days, so there are only memories and no physical evidence. It's for the best.

Three hours passed quickly. We delivered Penelope back to her waiting parents in the lobby. A few days later, Gloria appeared with a hand-written thank-you note.

"See?" she said. "You made her happy."

I was just relieved that the trauma gods had left us in peace.

Second Visit

Weeks later, Gloria reappeared in the doorway.

"Line 1. Penelope."

Gloria sat down again. She pointed at the speaker phone.

"Hi Dr. Buchman! I just wanted to tell you my report went great. Thank you again for letting me shadow you. It was amazing!"

Gloria crossed her arms, and I waited.

"I want to come back," Penelope continued. "My spring break is coming up, and my parents said it's okay to ask."

I scrawled a note to Gloria: ***This is a really bad idea***—underlining 'really' three times.

She merely smiled, gave me the "mom-look" and waved the thank-you note that had sat on my desk for nine months like my flag of surrender.

We set a date. That evening, after meeting Penelope and her parents, I led my new team in an unspoken prayer: Just a few calm hours, please.

The trauma gods were definitely not amused.

Moments later, digitals pagers on every belt erupted in unison, their harsh tones and scrolling numbers announcing a major trauma alert.

We raced to the bay, gowning and gloving as we entered.

A torrent of expletives presaged the arrival of a "DDGB-induced hyperacute lead poisoning", which was ED slang for "drug deal gone bad with a shootout." We counted three bullet holes. X-rays revealed a slug lodged in the left upper quadrant.

I asked a medical student to keep Penelope occupied while we operated. Please take her and keep her occupied in the cafeteria, library, anything.

The intern, resident, and I rolled the patient up to the OR. The anesthesiologist worked, the resident opened, and we found about a pint of blood and a bullet that had traversed the stomach and small bowel. The resident and I resected the injured bowel and put the ends back together. He was getting ready to close the stomach, but I stopped him and nodded toward the intern.

Surgery isn't a spectator sport. Learning happens the old way: see one, do one, teach one.

Stomach injuries are forgiving. Three layers of muscle in the stomach wall hold suture well. Those holes become good for teaching and good for learning. The senior resident stepped back. The intern took a breath and began. Her first stitch was tentative, but her second was confident. The repairs were beautiful.

I glanced at the clock. It was time to find the medical student and return Penelope to her parents. I asked the circulator to send out a page.

"No need," a voice said behind my left shoulder.

"…and I'm here over your right," added another.

Somehow, a high school freshman had made it into a trauma laparotomy.

The circulator shrugged. "What happens on night shift stays on night shift."

The scrub nurse winked.

The anesthesiologist did his best Sgt. Schulz impression: "I know nothing."

The operation had gone well. We delivered the patient to recovery and brought in the family. The intern glowed with pride; Penelope beamed with fascination.

We hustled her out of scrubs, found her parents in the lobby, and I explained Penelope's unexpected visit to the OR. They laughed. "Why did you think that was unexpected?"

Another handwritten thank-you arrived days later. Mission accomplished.

The Long Arc

The seasons turned and life at the hospital resumed its rhythm. One afternoon, as I was shrugging into my coat to go holiday shopping, Gloria appeared.

"Line 1. Penelope."

This time, she didn't bother with the speaker phone.

Penelope's visits became an annual ritual. She watched the new trauma center open, rode the elevator to the new helipad, and later went off to college. She applied to and entered medical school.

Today, she's an Assistant Professor. Her office is not far from the same lobby where we first met. She chose a specialty with a better work-life balance. She's married now, and herself a mom.

A quarter-century later, the rules have changed. No high-schoolers in the OR. Not ever.

That's fine; her specialty doesn't involve ORs.

Someday, though, her phone will ring. A tiny voice will say,

"I heard about you. I want to shadow you. It's for a school project."

And I hope she says yes.

Field Notes

The next generation arrives through primacy: the first rescue witnessed, the first mentor encountered, the first time someone is allowed to stand close enough to feel what rescue is.

Signal: When a trainee or a child asks, "Could I do that?" you are watching formation begin.

Failure modes: A thousand practical reasons to decline (time, policy, risk) can quietly become a habit of refusing access, and refusing access shrinks the pipeline.

Practice: Make mentorship concrete: offer a safe, bounded invitation; narrate what you are doing; let them carry one small responsibility. The goal is not to impress. The goal is to model what it feels like to serve.

DISCUSSION / WRITING PROMPTS (optional)

- What was the first rescue you witnessed, and what did it do to your sense of who you might become?
- Who was your first unforgettable mentor? What did they teach you that was not "content" but identity?
- When you are approached by a curious young person in uniform (on the street, in the hospital), what do you say about your work?

15 - STEEL

It was a September Sunday afternoon, usually a quiet shift. The knife-and-gun club was predictably asleep. The nearby interstate seemed sedate.

It seemed a good time to catch up on paperwork—or at least it was until the transfer center called about a helicopter inbound from a rural county sixty miles away.

"There's a bird in the air—ETA fifteen. They think you ought to meet them on the pad."

"What's up? Shock? Broken everything?"

"Doesn't sound like it. Vitals are normal, patient's talking. Guy in his forties."

"Then why the helicopter?"

"They said it's too complicated to explain."

Arrival

The helicopter settled onto the pad, rotors slowing. When the engine shut down, they waved me over.

The patient was awake, alert, and talking. That struck me as remarkable given that the patient had two feet of rebar—

steel reinforcing rod—running straight through his neck, with roughly nine inches protruding on either side.

He'd been riding his all-terrain vehicle near a construction site. The ATV went one way, the man went the other, and his neck met the rebar as he fell.

When he didn't return home, his family went looking for him. They found him lying sideways, steel through his neck, and called everyone they could think of: the volunteer ambulance, the volunteer fire department, and the sheriff's deputy.

They knew it would take a village.

The Village at Work

The first responders put their heads together.

The EMT and paramedic steadied his head while the firefighters found a saw powerful enough to cut the rebar.

The deputy cleared a landing zone and called in the helicopter.

Together they rolled him onto a short backboard so he could sit upright, improvising a way to stabilize his neck for flight.

Half an hour later, he was my patient. And I didn't have much more of a script than they did.

We rolled into the trauma bay and got the best X-rays we could manage, which wasn't saying much, since the view we really needed was blocked by the rebar itself.

A tetanus shot (we always gave them to penetrating trauma patients), some antibiotics, and then up to the OR.

The Sword and the Stone

The anesthesiologist took one look and said there was no way to place a breathing tube.

I told the man that I'd use numbing medication and place a temporary tracheostomy, a surgical airway that would stay in for a few days.

As I prepared, I heard rustling behind me. The flight crew had stayed, pulled on scrubs, and were now standing quietly, watching over my shoulder.

The trach went smoothly. The anesthesiologist connected the ventilator, and the man drifted off to sleep. I asked the scrub tech and resident to have a knife and vascular clamps ready.

I briefly wondered how King Arthur decided he was the one to pull the sword from the stone.

Then I pulled the rebar from the right side of his neck.

A Narrow Miss

Amazingly, there was no bleeding from the left side, and only a modest flow of venous blood from the right that I easily controlled with finger pressure.

I extended the incision and found a small branch of the jugular vein partially torn. Two clamps, a pair of silk ties, and the wound was dry. The rebar had missed every major vessel, slipped between the esophagus and the spine, and injured neither.

We irrigated both sides of the tract, placed drains, closed the wounds, and let the man surface gently from the anesthetic. He did astonishingly well. After a short recovery and confirmation that infection hadn't set in, we sent him home.

A few weeks later, he came back to the clinic, smiling, and we removed his tracheostomy tube. The staff had persuaded the pathologists to return the rebar. We had it cut into sections, each a few inches long. Removed the rust and the blood and had the sections sealed in some sort of clear plastic. Name and date on the plaques, each a memento of a warm September afternoon.

Rescues often take a village, improvisation, and several heaping tablespoons of luck. Fortunately, on that September afternoon, we had all three.

Field Notes

The trauma bay is the middle of the story, not the beginning. Rescue starts at the scene: access, extrication, hazards, and improvisation under constraint.

Signal: When the environment is unstable—traffic, fire, collapse, violence—scene safety and choreography become the first intervention.

Failure modes: Rushing to medical tasks before stabilizing the scene can injure rescuers and patients and can delay transport by creating secondary problems.

Practice: Build a mental checklist: scene safety, patient access, stabilization, packaging, and a clear handoff narrative that preserves what mattered before the lights of the bay.

DISCUSSION / WRITING PROMPTS (optional)

• What is the most complex or hazardous site you have had to work, and what made it safe enough to extract and transport?

• If you have managed an impalement, what principles guided your decisions? If you have not: what would you do first if you found someone impaled and unable to move?

16 - FROM ALIVE TO A LIFE

It was early evening, and I was rounding in the SICU when my BlackBerry buzzed with a text: Would I kindly stop by the medical intensive care unit and take a look at a patient? I crossed the elevator landing that divided the two ICUs. The MICU attending was concerned, and the family had somehow found my name and asked for me.

In the cubicle nearest the door lay a small woman, nearly hidden by her husband and sons. She was sixty years old. She had undergone a colon resection for recurrent diverticulitis. Such cases usually went well, except when they didn't.

This was one of those "didn't" cases. The patient also had polycystic kidney disease, and several of her cysts had begun leaking fluid into her abdomen, bathing the new bowel connection. Those reconnections (anastomoses) never seal immediately, even in the best of hands. Once bacteria found the warm fluid leaking from the cysts, they multiplied rapidly.

In medical terms, she was in septic shock. More simply, she had an infection that antibiotics could not clear, and her vital organs (her heart, blood vessels, kidneys, liver, lungs) were failing in sequence.

I called her surgeon. We reviewed two possibilities: she was either too sick to operate on or too sick not to be operated on. I persuaded the surgeon to bring out a colostomy, wash her out as best she could, and leave drains behind. A skilled anesthesiologist got her through the operation and back to the SICU. It was not a smooth course.

We adjusted her antibiotics. Her polycystic kidneys failed, and she required dialysis. She needed mechanical ventilation for weeks. She spent an entire season (three months) in the ICU before we could discharge her. After some time in rehab, she went home. She still needed two more operations: a colostomy reversal and a kidney transplant.

Months later, her husband called. She had stopped improving. There was no new infection, he told me, she had "just run out of gas". He said she was too weak for the surgeries that might restore her, yet unlikely to recover without them.

Alive, but with no prospects for life.

That call came late one afternoon as I was finishing a workout with my trainer, Diane. Her formal title is Medical Exercise Specialist. She watched my face fall as I listened. I explained to the patient's husband that this situation wasn't unusual. I could rescue and make someone "unsick", but it was beyond my power to make anyone "well".

When I hung up the call, Diane said something extraordinary:

"If you can get her to the gym, I'll do an assessment."

I called the husband back. The next day, the patient arrived. She was carried into the gym by her husband. She weighed seventy-eight pounds. She couldn't walk and could barely stand. Diane took a deep breath, helped her to her feet, and together they took three or four steps. That was all she could do, but Diane saw determination in her eyes.

"Your job," she told them, "is to get here. Mine is to help her move again."

They came every day. At six weeks, she had regained about 85% of her pre-sepsis strength. The surgeon performed the colostomy reversal. A month later, she was back in the gym.

A year later, the patient had another setback: pneumonia. One month in the hospital. Ten days after discharge, she was again in the gym. She was listed for a kidney transplant, which she received in 2008, twenty-seven months after I first met her. Back to the gym.

At three years, she was fully recovered. Her husband told me that she was back on the tennis court and winning matches. She lived another seventeen years. Diane continued to train her through early September 2025. Then came the final diagnosis: widely metastatic cancer. She died a few weeks later.

Her husband wrote to me after her death:

"I've told many people that your leadership of the SICU gave my wife twenty additional years. Thank you."

He was kind, but he was wrong.

It wasn't me.

It was Diane.

Diane and I shared several other patients during those years:

- A thirty-year-old medical student who was literally hit by a truck—sustaining head, chest, and abdominal injuries, as well as fractures in three of four limbs. I got her out of the hospital; Diane got her back to functioning. She finished medical school, matched into her first-choice residency, and today works for the federal government—a rock-star testament to the power of healing.

- A twenty-four-year-old lineman who touched a high-voltage wire; current arced through his arm and both legs. His heart stopped. CPR brought him back, but he suffered severe muscle injury and toe amputations. He left rehab barely able to walk. Diane took him on. Two decades later, he's fully functional—and works as a digital content creator.

- A thirty-four-year-old woman who sustained facial trauma and a shattered pelvis in a bicycle crash, complicated by venous thromboembolism. She hobbled on a walker, her legs swollen and painful. Diane worked with her for months. Years later, she returned to town—married, with a son—and still trains with Diane twice weekly.

- A twenty-two-year-old man who was ejected from a motor vehicle. His injuries filled a trauma textbook: closed head injury, pulmonary contusions, ruptured diaphragm, gastric laceration, and femoral fracture and dislocation. He left rehab on crutches, barely able to use them from profound muscle atrophy. Diane took him on. Today, he's a husband, father, and financial executive in the northeastern USA. He's fully functional, fully alive.

I kept them alive.

Diane gave them their lives back.

Some rescuers wear uniforms. Some wear scrubs.

And some, it turns out, wear polo shirts and count reps.

Field Notes

For rescuers, the rescue can feel like the end—paperwork done, the next call arrives. For patients, rescue is the beginning of a different life.

Signal: When the acute crisis resolves, the risk shifts from death to disability, despair, and the slow loss of function without a plan.

Failure modes: Treating rehabilitation as "someone else's problem" leaves patients without the second half of rescue: restoration of motion, meaning, and confidence.

Practice: Expand your definition of team. Find your 'Diane'—the body workers and rehabilitation experts who translate survival into a life worth living—and integrate them early, not as a late referral.

DISCUSSION / WRITING PROMPTS (optional)

• What is the most remarkable recovery you have witnessed, and who made it possible?

• How do you define functional outcome in your work (ADLs, strength, stamina, cognition, resilience)?

• Who belongs in your second circle of care (rehab, therapy, nutrition, social work, mental health), and how do you build reliable access to them?

17 - APPENDICITIS

Before appendectomy became the quintessential rite of passage for surgical trainees, it was the crucible through which modern clinical reasoning was forged. Its legacy begins with John P. Murphy, the Chicago surgeon who championed early operative intervention and described a canonical sequence of symptoms that medical students would memorize as "Murphy's March":

1. Periumbilical pain
2. Nausea, and vomiting
3. Migration of pain to the right lower quadrant
4. Fever
5. Leukocytosis

Each step in that progression corresponds to a distinct physiologic event. It begins with obstruction of a midgut hollow viscus—the appendix—stretching the visceral peritoneum and producing the vague, central pain of visceral distress. As inflammation extends to the parietal peritoneum, the pain localizes more sharply to the right lower quadrant. The later phases signal spillover of local inflammation to the body as a whole: fever and the surge of leukocytes.

Murphy's insight was more than descriptive; it was prescriptive. Each stage was both a warning and an opportunity. The clinician's task was to interrupt the march before it reached its terminal step, to act before rupture, before sepsis, before the patient's fate left the surgeon's hands.

We learned those steps long before CT scanners and ultrasound machines made appendicitis look obvious. Those "before times"—times before all-seeing technology told stories in pixels and voxels--demanded proximity to the patient, to one's own doubt, and to the anatomy beneath the skin.

We percussed gently, searching for the point of maximum tenderness. We tested for Rovsing's and psoas signs, watching for the flinch that told us the parietal peritoneum was inflamed. We squinted at plain abdominal films hoping to spot a faint appendicolith, a shadow of a stone in the right lower quadrant. Every finding was probabilistic; every decision, personal.

The ghost of John Murphy whispered to us all:
Don't let it rupture.

Teaching to Learn

I presided over hundreds of appendectomies, first as resident, then as a chief, and eventually as an attending surgeon. Most blurred together, but three on a single late-spring night in St. Louis remain vivid.

The gender mix of surgical training was changing, and that rotation I was blessed with an all-woman team: a senior resident, intern, and three medical students. They were bright, supportive, and full of mischief. The other services teased me about my entourage, a relic of an era before HR officers haunted the lounge, but the camaraderie was genuine.

One evening four cases came up from the ED. The first was a bowel obstruction, which was a perfect case for my senior resident to teach the intern while I stood back, holding retractors and still learning myself how to teach.

When that case was done, we called for the next patient and the first medical student. She approached expecting to hold retractors. Instead, I placed her on the right side of the table and whispered to the scrub tech:

"Knife to that doctor."

The tech grinned beneath his mask; he knew the play.

The first time one is trusted with a scalpel in the OR is an indelible event. *Me? Am I really ready?* I marked the umbilicus and anterior superior iliac spine, found McBurney's point, and drew the Rockey–Davis incision she had diagrammed days earlier on the whiteboard.

She opened the skin cleanly, then set the scalpel aside. The deeper layers yielded to Kelly clamps, not cuts. She spread the muscle fibers of the external, internal, and transversus abdominis, then tented the peritoneum with two forceps and nicked it gently with Metzenbaum scissors. A soft sigh of air entering the space. We—really, she—had entered the abdomen.

"Now," I said, "find a taenia and follow it down."

She took a Babcock clamp, found the taenia coli, and together we marched—one grasping, one releasing—until the base of the appendix came into view, inflamed and unmistakable.

"Make your index finger into a hook, and flip that worm up at me." She did, and I grabbed it with my Babcock.

"Good," I said. "Now two Kellys across the mesoappendix; divide between them -- scissors, not cautery. Ligate the appendiceal artery with 3-0 silk—snug, not strangling."

She did, perfect economy of motion.

"Next step," I said, "isn't the next step. Make a purse-string of 3-0 silk about a centimeter from the base. Then place a crushing clamp across the base, slide it half a centimeter toward the tip before the crush. Tie off the base with 3-0 chromic gut. Now amputate—scalpel along the underside of the clamp—and hand the appendix, clamp, and scalpel to the tech."

She followed each instruction flawlessly. Together we inverted the stump into the cecum as she cinched the purse-string closed.

We closed the peritoneum with 3-0 Vicryl, gently approximated the muscles and their fascia, finished with a subcuticular skin closure, and stepped back.

The anesthesiologist, lightening the anesthetic, looked up.

"Great job, doctor."

The student's eyes shined above her mask. Minutes later the patient was breathing on her own, transferred to the stretcher, and wheeled to recovery.

Later I heard she had dashed to the surgeons' lounge, picked up the phone, and whispered into the receiver, "*Hey Mom, are you awake? Guess what I just did!*"

Two more students. Two more appendices, gracefully liberated from the abdomens that held them. Two more calls to moms. The night had completed its teaching.

Learning to Teach

One of those students became a general surgeon, beginning her own list of appendices that would be learned and taught.

Another became an internist.

The third became a psychiatrist.

Four years later an email arrived:

"*Dear Dr. Buchman,*

You might not remember a night when three medical students each took out an appendix.

You might think the lesson was... well... wasted on a psychiatrist-to-be.

But out here in the Rocky Mountains, you made a difference.

This morning the nurses told me that a patient on our locked ward had been vomiting all night. I examined him and he was quite tender at McBurney's point.

'He has appendicitis,' I said. They were dubious at best. Patients don't get appendicitis on a psychiatric service. We don't usually perform abdominal exams.

But I did.

I remembered our patient and what that appendix looked like.

We called surgery.

They took him to the OR.

It was indeed appendicitis."

Another rescue. I read it twice, then smiled. Her experience had traveled farther than either of us expected.

Coda

Today, CT scans can diagnose appendicitis with near-certainty, and clinical trials debate whether antibiotics might replace surgery altogether. Yet technology cannot replicate what those long nights taught us: that anatomy and pathology must be felt, not merely seen; that judgment is built in layers (like the abdominal wall itself) and that teaching and learning are reciprocal acts.

We learn to teach by giving away what was once hard-won. We teach to learn by watching another's hands discover what our own once feared. Between the two lies the enduring art of surgery. Underlying all, though, is the satisfaction of rescue.

Field Notes

Teaching rescue is engineered autonomy: high standards, honest feedback, and progressive responsibility without making failure obligatory.

Signal: The apprenticeship relationship is itself a clinical instrument: when it works well, both patient safety and trainee growth improve.

Failure modes: Unclear expectations, inconsistent feedback, and humiliation-as-teaching produce either timid trainees or reckless ones. Both are unsafe.

Practice: Set stretch goals with guardrails. Mix the expected with the unexpected. Normalize questions. Make debriefs routine. And remember: you cannot predict what a trainee will carry for decades—so teach with care.

DISCUSSION / WRITING PROMPTS (optional)

• What lesson stayed with you for years and then resurfaced unexpectedly? What made it stick?

• What feedback have apprentices given you that changed how you teach (or how you lead) afterward?

18 - T(ERROR)

Every surgeon makes errors.

With time we develop better judgment, better choosing the right operation for the right patient at the right moment. Our technical skills sharpen; our tissue handling grows more deliberate; our instincts improve. Yet no matter how seasoned we become, there are days when our skill, judgment, or simple human limitation collides with the chaos of injury. Sometimes we make serious errors. We make many. I have made many.

This is the story of one of mine.

A major trauma alert had been called for a teenager shot in the right flank. Pale, sweaty, tachycardic, hypotensive. He was losing blood fast. There was no time for deliberation. He needed the operating room, and he needed it now.

Anesthesia induced. More IVs. Antiseptic, drapes, clips. A long midline incision. At once, blood welled up from the abdomen. The source, however, hid itself.

There are parts of the torso that are friendly, and parts that are decidedly not. That morning we found ourselves entering one of the most unforgiving: the central retroperitoneum, where the largest vessels of the body run deep, guarded by spinal column behind and major viscera ahead and to either side. No surgeon ventures there casually. But this morning we had no choice. Blood was pouring out, and the only path to stop the bleeding and perform a rescue was through it.

Forceps, scissors, spongesticks for pressure. Suction slurping blood as fast as it appeared. The chief resident and I worked in a synchronized frenzy while the anesthesiologist transfused four units, then six, then eight. Fifteen minutes later we had controlled the major bleeding. One pulverized kidney had to be removed. We irrigated the blood away and studiously revisited the bullet's path, searching for any undetected injuries left in its wake.

We found one that wasn't the bullet's.

A few minutes into this "what else is injured here" look-see, I recognized a devastating sight: I had inadvertently divided and ligated the vein draining the patient's other kidney.

Without that vein, the remaining kidney would swell, congest, and die. He would be consigned to a life on a dialysis machine.

There is no horror quite like the moment one realizes that one has injured a patient—not abstractly, not "in theory," but concretely, undeniably, through one's own hand. It did not matter that we were operating in a distorted field. It did not matter that we were fighting to save his life. All that mattered was that I had caused a new, potentially catastrophic problem.

There is no checklist for this moment. No algorithm for how to manage one's own fear and shame while continuing to operate. All we have is the obligation to do the next right thing and do it right now. At that moment, I was looking at a warm kidney with a severed vein.

Years of rotation through vascular, transplant, and trauma services had given me a mental map of how surgeons handle kidneys *in extremis*. I recognized what I was looking at: a step in a kidney transplant, only not in context.

I did two things.

First, I prepared the kidney as if it were about to be transplanted. Surgeons know not to make stuff up, rather to do things that work. Indeed, that is the secret to most unexpected situations-transform the problem into something seen before, and follow in others' footsteps. I clamped the artery to prevent swelling. Infused cold preservative solution. Packed cold slush around the organ to slow its metabolism.

Second, and far more important, I asked the circulator to page the transplant surgeon on call and to please tell him I needed him right now.

He arrived within minutes. I met him at the door and said plainly what had happened, what I had done, and what I needed.

"No problem," he said.

He scrubbed, gowned, joined me at the table. Together we dissected the ends of the injured vein. Then, with a calm that only comes from deep mastery, he reattached the kidney's vein to a draining vein in the patient.

Twelve more minutes. That was all it took.

I thanked him. He left. The kidney pinked up and continued working perfectly.

Weeks later, I presented the case at Morbidity and Mortality conference, the regular gathering where surgeons review complications, confess misjudgments, and commit to doing better. After I described the case, the chair invited the transplant surgeon to speak.

He began by gently but firmly rebuking me for causing the injury. I deserved it. Then he turned to the room and did something else entirely.

He said that because I had quickly preserved the kidney, and because I had stepped back from pride and called for help, the patient suffered neither morbidity nor mortality. This case, he said, was simply a brief misadventure with a happy ending. Then, in full view of the trainees, he came to the podium, shook my hand, and said that knowing when to ask a colleague for assistance was an essential mark of surgical mastery.

In the end, the patient did well.

So did his surgeon.

Error is part of rescue. Any rescuer who works long enough carries memories of decisions or actions they wish they could rewrite. I have so many that they could easily fill another book. But this chapter is about something deeper than error.

It is about the truth that none of us rescues alone.

Calling for help is not an admission of weakness.

It is not merely humility.

It is an intervention.

It protects the patient.

It protects the rescuer.

And sometimes, as in this case, it saves an organ, a life, and a future.

In rescue, asking for help is itself an act of rescue.

Rescuer In The Mirror

Sooner or later, every rescuer harms someone. Sometimes it is error. Sometimes it is misadventure. Sometimes it is the unavoidable injury created by the very intervention meant to save. When it happens, the reflex is to shrink, hide, and try to outrun the moment with speed.

But the moment demands two rescues: the patient's and yours. The patient needs immediate stabilization, a broader brain at the bedside, and a plan that is no longer solo. You need containment, honesty, and a path through shame before shame starts making decisions for you.

My advice: rehearse this before it happens. When harm occurs: stop the bleeding (literal or metaphorical), call for help early, state the facts plainly, and accept assistance without bargaining for your image. Debrief the event, document it, and use the supports offered—peer review, morbidity-and-mortality, counseling—because you cannot practice safely while carrying untreated injury inside yourself.

Your memories of what went wrong will never entirely leave. They will return, ghostlike—sometimes while caring for another patient, sometimes in a dream, sometimes in those moments where the water is cascading over you while rinsing away sins real and imagined.

Mirror question: If you caused harm today, who is the first person you would call? Why that person?

19 - THE HOLIDAY CARD

Autumn Into Winter, Present Day

In the quiet days after last Thanksgiving—now nearly four decades into hearing Mariah Carey assure us that "All I Want for Christmas Is You"—the first holiday cards began to arrive. The usual assortment fills the mailbox: corporate bulk mailings, the "remember us" appeals from charitable organizations, and the end-of-year catch-ups from colleagues, friends, and family. Each year, Barbara opens and sorts them, arranging the most colorful along the credenza behind our dining room table: red and green here, blue and white there.

And then there is the card.

One envelope she always sets aside. She recognizes the return address instantly. She knows what's inside: a simple card on heavy stock, a photograph of a handsome couple surrounded by their children. High-school sweethearts, now adults with large lives. He has risen to become a Managing Director at a financial services firm with a name everyone knows.

I met them long before any of that. I met them on a spring day late in the last century, when they were college students planning a wedding.

A Saturday in Springtime, Late 1990s

The trauma pager sounded, summoning the team to the bay. We were receiving victims from a horrific car crash. The vehicle, a 1987 Cadillac Coupe DeVille, offered shoulder belts and airbags for the front seats. The rear seats, though, had only lap belts of the same style you still find on many commercial airliners.

You likely know the airliner safety briefing by heart: "Fasten the belt low and tight across your hips."

That admonition is written in blood.

When a vehicle suddenly decelerates, the body keeps moving forward. In those first milliseconds, every tissue behind a poorly positioned belt is driven against bone. Over the pelvis, there is little to compress. Across the abdomen, where belts so often rest casually fastened near the navel, the consequences are catastrophic.

First comes compression: abdominal wall, bowel, and great vessels all forced back against the spine.

Then comes rotation: the mass of the unrestrained torso pitching forward, continuing its doomed trajectory toward the windshield.

The result is shear: tissue tearing from tissue, vessel from vessel.

Trauma surgeons shorten the entire explanation to three words: lap belt injury.

The outward clue may be a faint bruise. The inward reality is devastation.

The high-school sweethearts, now college students, had been sitting together in the back seat. They had done what the car offered: buckled the lap belts.

The Trauma Bay

Their gurneys arrived in tandem and veered into adjoining rooms. The team leaders began their practiced fugue across the doorway:

"Airway, Breathing, Circulation, Disability, Exposure."

"Talk to me—what's your name? Deep breath. Again. Don't move; that's an IV."

"Wiggle your fingers and toes while we cut off your clothes."

Trauma shears sliced through spring cotton. Under the lights, the hidden truths emerged.

"Secondary survey."

"Lap-belt sign, distended, tender abdomen."

An echo in the next room:

"Secondary survey. Lap-belt bruise, rigid abdomen."

Both needed the operating room. But who first?

Amid their pleas for us to care for the other, we confronted the unlovely calculus of trauma:

Which injury might be simpler? and therefore faster to fix?

Should we summon the on-call team, knowing it would take an hour?

Should we take the more complex case first and hope the other did not suddenly collapse?

And what of the inevitable next patient already *en route*?

General Omar Bradley famously remarked:
"Amateurs talk about strategy. Professionals talk about logistics."
In trauma, we talk about both.

The labs returned with a sinister refrain: A, B, C.
Acidosis, Bleeding, Coagulopathy.
My patients looked better than they were.

Damage control was the only path: stop the bleeding, stop the leaking, wash out the abdomen, restore warmth.

Time to move.

The Operating Room

They were trauma twins now, their injuries parallel but not equal. His were worse.

I am reminded here of Omar Khayyam:
"When I want to understand what is happening today, or try to decide what will happen tomorrow, I look back."

To understand his devastation, one must look back to his mother's womb, late in the first trimester. The embryo destined to become the future Managing Director was then four or five centimeters long. His intestines, already lengthening and branching, had herniated into the umbilical cord to grow outside the body. Picture a leaf: its stem fixed to the spine, its vascular lacework fanning outward. Over weeks, it lengthened, folded, rotated 270 degrees, and returned to the abdominal cavity. This exquisitely delicate network would nourish him for the rest of his life.

Until the crash.

When the lap belt struck, some loops of bowel burst outright, releasing gas and chyme into the abdomen. Others were pinned against the spine as their fragile vascular stems stretched and snapped, leaving segments that looked deceptively healthy but were fatally devascularized.

His Operation

Opening his abdomen revealed chaos: frothy fluid, clotted blood, shredded mesentery. The story of blunt force was written in every direction.

Some bowel was clearly dead; some looked nearly normal but could not be trusted. We resected what was unquestionably nonviable. The borderlands where viability remained uncertain would declare themselves with time.

We stapled off ends of bowel, avoiding reconnection. We irrigated, warmed, controlled bleeding, packed the abdomen, and sent him to the ICU.

Only a second look would reveal how much bowel might survive.

Her Operation

Next door, her abdomen told a different story.

Her intestinal injuries were limited to a few contusions, abrasions, and a few short devascularized segments of no immediate danger.

Her major injury was to the abdominal wall itself.

All three layers of the musculature (the rectus, obliques, and transversus) had been shredded. Not cut or torn: delaminated. Muscle stripped from fascia, fascia from peritoneum, entire layers peeled apart by a force that behaved more like a blunt guillotine than a restraint.

You cannot sew shredded muscle as if it were cloth. You cannot restore blood supply to dead fibers. Reconstruction becomes a negotiation with biology.

We controlled bleeding, removed what was nonviable, restored what continuity we could, and accepted the rest would declare itself with time.

The Night Between

In the ICU the trauma twins lay in adjacent rooms again, separated by a wall but bound by catastrophe. They fought the triad—cold, acidosis, coagulopathy. We rewarmed, repleted, and stabilized.

But for him, one question hovered:

How much bowel is alive?

No surgeon knows the answer after the first operation. Only the tissue knows.

We planned the second look for the next day.

Second Looks — The Reckoning

Second-look operations are courtroom dramas. The abdomen is reopened; last night's packing removed; the viscera separated by fresh white sponges.

And then we call an expert witness and his tool.

Robert Williams Wood—physicist, inventor of the black light. And fluorescein—a xanthene dye that glows yellow-green where blood still flows.

We dried all surfaces. The anesthesiologist injected fluorescein. We waited twelve minutes. The circulator darkened the room.

The Wood's lamp came on.

Where fluorescein had traveled, the bowel glowed green. Where the lamp revealed only blackness, the tissue was dead.

His intestine remained mostly dark.

We marked the margins, restored the lights, and cut away what would not sustain him. What remained would never be enough. Should he survive, he would live with short-gut syndrome for the rest of his days.

The physics of an instant had become the calculus of a lifetime.

Weeks Later

They survived. Partners in suffering, they handed each other forward. When one faltered, the other steadied. Alongside our nurses and therapists, they bonded with the three specialists essential to his future: the pharmacist, the nutrition support specialist, and the dietitian. Together they orchestrated the intricate daily mimicry of the small intestine, delivering nutrients, vitamins, electrolytes, and water directly to his bloodstream.

Even after discharge, they remained at his side. I saw them all in clinic, but the long healing belonged to this remarkable little circle.

Another Spring Saturday, Three Years Later

A wedding invitation arrived.

The ceremony joined not only two beautiful young people, but two survivors and all who had accompanied them. In the photographs, the happiest faces may have been those flanking the couple: the surgeon, the dietitian, the nutrition support specialist, and the pharmacist. We were there not to rescue but to witness.

For years, the photograph hung in the ICU where they had once fought for their lives. Staff passed it daily, a reminder of why we do this work. Eventually, the ICU moved to a newer, brighter space, and the photograph began its own journey.

Autumn Into Winter, Present Day

The holiday card—the one with the photo of a handsome couple and their children—smiled from our credenza through the New Year. Each year, when Barbara decides it is time to return the ornaments and star to the security of their tissue-paper nests in the basement, it falls to me to clear the credenza and carry the cards to recycling.

There is always that one card at the top of the stack.

I descend to the lower level, cards in hand. From the kitchen above me comes once more the unmistakable sound of "All I Want for Christmas Is You". It will be the last time I listen to it until next November.

In the basement corridor, I pause.

I hold this year's card—husband, wife, three beautiful children all a year older now—up to a framed wedding photograph taken a quarter-century ago. The young couple, the four of us flanking them, all smiles, all promise.

The image has not aged; only we have.

Rescues belong to the rescued, not the rescuer.

They live in the lives that continue, and in the families that flourish.

The annual card is merely the reminder. It is an echo from the past, renewed each year like the perennial return of that familiar holiday song.

Mariah reaches her final refrain as I turn back up the stairs. I have my memories. They have their rescue.

It is their rescue that endures.

Rescuer In The Mirror

Time turns rescues into memory.

Patients go on, and we go on, and most of what remains is an internal archive: names, faces, and the quiet realization that the wheel of rescue keeps turning whether we are watching it or not.

Still, some rescues resurface with artifacts—a card, a photograph, a message years later. They are not trophies. They are proof that downstream life exists, and that our work sometimes echoes farther than we will ever know.

My advice: hold on to those names and those moments without claiming ownership of them. Rescues belong to the rescued. But their gratitude, when it arrives, can become balm—an antidote to cynicism and a reminder that your place on each turn of the wheel has meaning.

Mirror question: What artifact of gratitude are you willing to let yourself receive without deflecting it?

20 - CURTAIN CALL

Perhaps you circle dates on the family refrigerator calendar. Perhaps you assign yourself a special color on your smartphone. Perhaps you let your digital assistant remind you.

Tomorrow you are **on**.

Your shift begins at some ungodly hour. You and your uniform, the tools and badges that identify you must be clean, polished, and ready to serve.

You have spent days and weeks and months—and perhaps years, even decades—preparing for your next shift.

Nothing quite prepares you for your last.

The signals arrive quietly. You have your pick of the schedule. Novices gravitate toward you, eager for war stories and wisdom. The service pin on your lapel is no longer ten-year bronze, or even twenty-year silver. You wear your thirty-year gold with pride, though it has become harder to read in dim light and without eyeglasses.

If you are a first responder, a party might be scheduled. You've attended enough such heartfelt tributes with laughter. Speeches that are half roast, half blessing. A slideshow made from faded snapshots pulled from family albums. A name added to an honor roll. A gift meant to bridge an adrenaline-drenched day into a different kind of evening. A toast.

And then there is a call. Gear is grabbed. The vehicle rolls without you.

If you are a senior professor in an academic center, there might be an event. If you are a trauma surgeon or an ICU doctor, there might be a retelling of this or that spectacular "save." Your successor offers homilies and reassurance that the work you started will continue.

If you are an academic leader, there might be an easel and a canvas, your gaze destined to grace some wall in some hallway on some floor in a building somewhere in the complex. There is a hollow invitation to "stop by anytime," and a last handshake.

In the distance a siren wails. Instead of the rush to the ED, there is the walk to the parking lot.

For most of us, that is the end.

For a very few, there is one more curtain call.

In the middle of the twentieth century, professional societies of creatives popularized the Lifetime Achievement Award—an honor for careers of sustained effort, excellence, and influence, a visible acknowledgment of a fulfilled professional journey. These curtain calls serve several purposes: to acknowledge a past, to inspire a future, to catalyze donations for a current cause. There is remembrance—an exhibition, an invited lecture, something to celebrate the giant whose shoulders are yet visible, at least to those who stand on them.

Still, it is a last curtain call. And more than a few of the audience who saw or knew or stood have already left the theatre when it is your final turn to take the stage.

You will have noticed that these lifetime achievement awards are doled out very sparingly—often not more than one each year. The selection process is uneasy, even in the early years of a professional society. Later, it becomes much more difficult.

I chaired such a selection committee two decades ago, when my professional society of rescuers was yet young. I read the endorsements and listened to the passions advocating for this or that candidate. Each was worthy. Yet only one could be forwarded to the board. The rest would receive a lovely letter explaining that it was an honor in itself to be considered.

Two Years Ago

A couple of years ago, a sponsor came to me and asked for my CV. It was time, they said lovingly, for someone to advocate for me.

In due course, they sent me a nominating letter for proofreading. It was the sort of letter that makes parents blush. I would have shared it with mine, but they too had already left this earthly stage somewhere in the final act of my professional life.

A few days later, I got a call. Another very worthy candidate was also being proposed, and would I do them the honor of writing *their* nominating letter?

They did not know I was also a candidate.

This other candidate, nearly a decade older than me, had also had an illustrious and meaningful career. Present nearly at the creation of our discipline. A classic trajectory of hard work that led to international leadership. A model for others to emulate. A grace with no parallel among our ranks.

I could have demurred.

Instead, I said it would be my honor to pen the letter.

The letter, more than three single-spaced pages, would have made their parents blush. But their parents had also left the earthly theatre a decade before mine.

I closed my letter with these words, a sort of solo *pas de deux*:

> "The nominee is now nearly eight decades on this planet. As Geoffrey Chaucer remarked in *The Clerk's Tale*:
>
> *'For thogh we slepe, or wake, or rome, or ryde, Ay fleeth the tyme; it nyl no man abyde.'*
>
> (For though we sleep, or wake, or roam, or ride, time will fly; it will pause for no man.)

I do not know how many more opportunities the professional society will have to honor the nominee with the Lifetime Achievement Award. I urge the selection committee to make this year the nominee's year."

A Few Months Later

A few months later, I received three notes in quick succession.

The first told me that although I did not receive the award, it was a great honor to even be nominated.

The second told me that my letter had carried the day for the other candidate.

The third was from the other candidate, joyful, grateful, inviting me to the celebration.

Not long after, my younger advocate who had labored so hard to write a nominating letter on my behalf spoke with me.

"You sort of sandbagged yourself," she grumbled. It was the gentlest of grumbles, yet a grumble nonetheless.

We spoke for a time, and I saw a glimmer of understanding in her eyes. Rescue, I said, is not so much about what we do as what we are about. In the end, whether it be at the end of a case, a shift, a year, or a lifetime, we are about making someone else's life a little better.

It's not just the older person who has fallen, or the child with an allergic reaction, or the family stuck in the ditch when their car ran off the road. It is each other. Because eventually we or someone we love will be that older person, or that child, or that family.

The Next Cycle

The seasons changed, and another nominations cycle came. My young advocate sent the letter back in, revised to include a gentle reference to the prior year's ballet. There was not even a hint of grumble.

A few weeks ago, I received a single letter. It began, "*Congratulations on being selected as the recipient of the Lifetime Achievement Award...*"

I sent a note to my advocate, and she is just as thrilled as she would have been the prior year.

The ceremony and my lecture lies a year in the future. This book that you hold is a step in my preparation towards this curtain call, a quiet affirmation of the gift of being on this path of rescue.

Epilogue - The Privilege of Endless Rescue

And the end of all our exploring
Will be to arrive where we started
And know the place for the first time.
— T. S. Eliot, Little Gidding

There comes a point in every rescuer's life when the question "*Why am I on this path?*" quietly transforms into "*Where does this path lead?*"

At first, the answer feels tangible: toward competence, redemption, mastery. Toward some imagined horizon where the debts of the past are finally paid and there will be peace with what has been done and left undone.

That horizon never arrives. The rescuer discovers that the path loops back on itself, an unending circuit of calls, responses, losses, and small salvations. The work is never done because the rescuer's world is never whole. Each success reveals another fracture; each reprieve expires at dawn.

It seems like futility; in fact, it is our shared grace.

The Thermodynamics of Service

Like the laws that govern the physical world, the rescuers' moral universe has its own thermodynamics. Here are our rules:

- We can't win. Every rescue is temporary; the next crisis awaits.
- We can't break even. The debts of love, duty, and care grow with each encounter.
- And we can't get out of the game. To live is to engage, to re-enter the field again and again.

Yet within those limits lies meaning.

The endless cycle is not punishment; it is participation in the fundamental exchange of life. Eventually the lesson becomes clear: that to work within limits is to join the great current of compassion that flows through generations.

What endures is not victory, but continuity.

The Transformation of Understanding

In the beginning, each rescue feels like a challenge. Each feels like a test of your knowledge and skill, of your courage and will. With time and complications, you sense that rescue is an illumination of the limit dividing what we can and cannot do, each rescue tinged with penance for old failures and helplessness. Only with time does it mature into comprehension: a steady, wordless knowing that the act of returning itself is the redemption.

To rescue again is to affirm that meaning is made, not found. The endless repetition of service becomes its own revelation: this is what it means to be human—fragile, flawed, yet faithful to the end.

Recalling past cases stirs memories of sadness and of joy. They are not opposites but companions, moving in tandem through the circular path. Sadness for what could not be kept; joy for what can still be given.

The Covenant of the Rescuer

Those who answer the call to rescue join an ancient covenant. It is that quiet promise heard from those who came before that we now whisper to those we train. Perhaps you think it differently, perhaps you express it differently, but it is the same, and it always has been the same. These words have guided me, and surely they resonate with you:

You will not win, but you will matter.
You will not be remembered, but you will belong.
You will not find rest, but you will find meaning.

To choose this life of rescue is to accept that belonging is more precious than victory. To stand in the stream of suffering and keep your footing, to steady another life for a moment, is to participate in something larger than self.

Here is the truth that every rescuer at peace with themselves has learned: *we were never here to be redeemed, but to reveal what redemption looks like.*

The Privilege of Beginning Again

Eliot was right: the end of all our exploring will be to arrive where we started and know the place for the first time. We return to each new beginning—the pager's call, the siren, the dark hallway—but now with open eyes. We see the cycle for what it is: not a trap, but rather a testament.

Every faith tradition teaches its own version of this truth, our truth. In Judaism, it is written in the Mishnah: "He who saves a single life saves all mankind." In the Qur'an, it is echoed almost word for word. Christian teaching calls the rescuer to see the divine in "the least of these." Buddhism speaks of the bodhisattva's vow never to abandon the suffering world. Hinduism, of seva—selfless service—as the highest form of devotion. Each, in its own tongue and rhythm, recognizes that to preserve life is to participate in the sacred act of creation itself.

This is the ecumenical sanctification of every rescuer. It spans creed and uniform, license and credential. It arises at every station on the arc of care, in every person who stands between chaos and another's end. You become their shield, stare into their abyss and in your role and with your skill say, "*Not now, not yet.*"

Grace

The rescuer's grace – your grace -- is never found in a single shimmering instant, but in repeated glimpses of something more wondrous: each flash of coherence in the midst of disorder, each moment a breath returns, each pause of shared silence after crisis, each a knowing look among the weary who have done what they could today and will do it again tomorrow. Each glimpse is both ephemeral and eternal, evidence that, despite all our limits, you and I have been gifted the privilege of touching what is infinite.

So our work – yours and mine -- goes on. We do not get out of the game; rather, we are grateful to remain in it. In each new beginning, we are reminded that the practice of truth, like this practice of rescue, was never about reaching the end, but about recognizing the holiness of beginning again.

My exit is just ahead, my off-ramp from this wheel of rescue. I am glad to know it is there and I will be glad to be taking it. I have been absorbed into the braid that the wheel spins off, a thread in this braid of rescuers that goes back millennia and will extend to the end of days.

Acknowledgements

The through-line of this book—*No one rescues alone*—applies equally to its making.

No one writes alone.

My reinvention from academic clinician-scientist to author and speaker would not have been as smooth or as rewarding without the advice, reassurance, and gentle prodding of my editor, Tammy Kling, and my mentor, Bethany Williams. Their insight, candor, and generosity continue to shape both the work and the worker. I look forward to their counsel in the years ahead. Put simply, the publication of this book marks the *end of the beginning* of my reinvention. The book may be finished; I am not. My thanks also to Harry Greenspun, the colleague who first connected me with these remarkable women.

Ernest Hemingway famously observed that "all first drafts are [expletive]." To those who endured mine with patience and sharpened the later ones with precision—Katie Casey, Nancy Chambers, Diane Dito, Wendy Feign, Bob Hannaford, Sheila Owen, Paul Pepe, Laura Pooler, Steve Simpson, and Tammie Quest, thank you. (I'll thank Nancy Chambers one more time for her careful final proofreading.) You made this book better. More importantly, your friendship over the years has made me better.

The stories told here are all true. Each patient's experience is presented in anonymous third person, but every one of them remains vivid and dear to me. As for the rescuers, some are named—with their consent. When I reached out to ask whether they preferred real names or pseudonyms, I was deeply moved by their unanimous encouragement. They wanted these stories told for the same reason I wanted to tell them: because their meaning reaches beyond the medical record.

Of course, not every story could be included. This is a memoir, not an encyclopedic record. Still, I have been formed and guided by my time at The University of Chicago, The Johns Hopkins Medical Institutions, Shock Trauma (MIEMSS), Washington University in St. Louis (Barnes-Jewish Hospital), and my current academic home, Emory University and Emory Healthcare, as well as by colleagues across many professional societies. Where you find success in these pages, the credit is largely theirs; where things went sideways, the responsibility is mine alone.

Finally, something more than an acknowledgement.

I met my wife, Barbara, more than fifty-one years ago —she was my teacher in medical school. She has lived every story in this book, not as rescuer but as my anchor and on more than one occasion, as my savior. She and our daughter Rachel (whose byline I am immensely proud to read) have been there for me, waited for me, laughed with me, and now look back with me. Whatever light shines from these pages, I am just a reflector. My light comes from them.

Chestnut Hall Books publishes thoughtful works shaped by experience, integrity, and a commitment to truth.

Each book is written to serve—offering counsel, perspective, and practical wisdom that supports readers in life, work, and meaningful endeavor.

CHESTNUT HALL
BOOKS

www.ingramcontent.com/pod-product-compliance
Lightning Source LLC
LaVergne TN
LVHW010659110826
845149LV00014B/3159
* 9 7 9 8 9 9 5 1 3 2 8 0 6 *